PROFESSIONAL LIABILITY AND RISK MANAGEMENT

A Resource for
Obstetrician–Gynecologists
in Training and in Practice

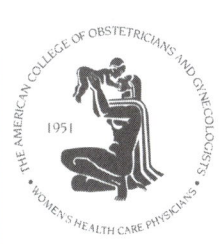

The American
College of
Obstetricians
and
Gynecologists

*Women's Health
Care Physicians*

Professional Liability and Risk Management: A Resource for Obstetrician–Gynecologists in Training and in Practice was developed under the direction of the Committee on Professional Liability:
Willette L. LeHew, MD, FACOG, Chair
Larry L. Veltman, MD, FACOG, Vice Chair
Erol Amon, MD, JD, FACOG
Victoria L. Green, MD, JD, FACOG
Johanna F. Perlmutter, MD, FACOG
Steven D. Wolf, DO, FACOG

Department of Professional Liability/Risk Management Staff
Albert L. Strunk, JD, MD, FACOG, Vice President, Fellowship Activities Division
Sharon Kenyon, RN, JD, Associate Director, Department of Professional Liability/Risk Management
Linda Esser, Administrator, Projects and Research
Charlene Burger, Administrative Assistant

The information in *Professional Liability and Risk Management: A Resource for Obstetrician–Gynecologists in Training and in Practice* provides risk management information that is current as of the date issued and is subject to change. This document does not define a standard of care nor should it be interpreted as legal advice. As always, physicians should consult their personal attorneys about legal requirements in their jurisdictions and for legal advice on particular matters.

Referral to Internet sites does not imply the endorsement of the American College of Obstetricians and Gynecologists. References to such web sites are not meant to be comprehensive; the exclusion of a web site does not reflect the quality of that web site. Please note that web sites and uniform resource locators are subject to change without warning. Many of these pages provide basic information but have links with more detailed information and resources.

Copyright © 2002 by the American College of Obstetricians and Gynecologists

Library of Congress Cataloging-in-Publication Data

Professional liability and risk management: a resource for obstetrician-gynecologists in training and in practice/developed under the direction of the Committee on Professional Liability.
  p. cm
Includes bibliographical references and index.
ISBN 0-915473-84-4 (alk. paper)
  1. Gynecologists--Malpractice--United States. 2. Obstetricians--Malpractice--United States. I. American college of Obstetricians and Gynecologists. Committee on Professional Liability.
KF2910.G943 P768 2002
344.73'04121--dc21

2002003452

12345/65432

Contents

Preface   vii

Chapter 1   The Elements of Professional Liability   1

Duty   2
Breach of Duty   5
Causation   5
Damages   6

Chapter 2   The Stages of a Medical Professional Liability Lawsuit—Pretrial Stage   7

Incident Management   8
Notice of a Claim   9
Discovery Procedures   11
Depositions   13

Chapter 3   The Stages of a Medical Professional Liability Lawsuit—Trial Stage   19

Being an Effective Witness at Trial   20
Trial   22

Chapter 4   The Stages of a Medical Professional Liability Lawsuit—Settlement Stage   27

Mediation   28
Factors Influencing the Decision to Settle   30
Settlement of an Incident   31
Settlement of a Formal Claim or Lawsuit   31

CHAPTER 5   Informed Consent   33

   Degree of Disclosure   35
   State Laws on Informed Consent   38
   The Process of Informed Consent   38
   Informed Refusal   40
   Informed Consent Forms   41

CHAPTER 6   Risk Management Issues   43

   Risk Management in the Hospital Setting   44
   Risk Management in the Outpatient/Ambulatory Care Setting   47

CHAPTER 7   Special Liability Issues for Residents   51

   Liability Status   52
   Ethical Considerations   56

CHAPTER 8   High-Risk Areas for Litigation in Obstetrics
   and Gynecology   59

   The Neurologically Impaired Infant   61
   Delivery Methods   61
   Shoulder Dystocia   63
   Breast Cancer   63
   Other Areas of High Risk   65

CHAPTER 9   Patient Communication   67

CHAPTER 10   Medical Records   71

   Accuracy   73
   Comprehensiveness   73
   Legibility   74
   Objectivity   75
   Timeliness   75
   Correcting Medical Records   76

CHAPTER 11   Professional Liability Insurance   79

   Professional Liability Insurance Coverage During Residency   80
   Professional Liability Insurance Coverage After Residency   85

CHAPTER 12 Examples of Government Requirements
Affecting Medical Practice   91

   Patient Screening and Transfer (Emergency Medical Transfer
      in Active Labor Act)   92
   Privacy and Accountability of Individually Identifiable Health
      Information   95
   Fraud and Abuse   97
   Medical Office Environment   98

CHAPTER 13 Physician Reporting Requirements and
Profiling   101

   The Data Banks   102
   State Physician Profiling   106

References   107

Glossary   109

   Medical–Legal Terms   109
   Professional Liability Insurance Definitions and Terms   118

Index   121

Preface

Current obstetric and gynecologic practice has become part of an increasingly complex health care delivery system in which physicians are likely to encounter medical–legal issues directly affecting their own practices or the practices of their colleagues. The reality of the medical–legal interface must be understood in relation to, among other things, the process of litigation, informed consent, patient communication, and medical record keeping. Because each of these represents the potential for professional liability, it is imperative that residents and, indeed, all physicians, learn the basic elements of risk management. As stated in the CREOG Educational Objectives, Seventh Edition: "…residents-in-training must become aware of the clinical events that most commonly precipitate malpractice claims and develop strategies to minimize the risk of such claims." Moreover, physicians must "…understand the sequence of events associated with a malpractice suit and adopt coping mechanisms to lessen the impact of such a suit on their practices and their families."

The Department of Professional Liability/Risk Management and the Committee on Professional Liability undertook the revision of this resource to provide residents and practicing obstetrician–gynecologists with basic concepts regarding issues in professional liability and risk management. Although the purpose of this document is not scientific in nature or focus, it is relevant to the practice of medicine in our present culture. Accordingly, each chapter stands alone to highlight key areas, and collectively they serve as a source of information that can be used to help resident physicians, as well as all physicians in clinical practice, prepare for the challenges of practicing obstetrics and gynecology in a litigation-oriented society.

This document is not meant to be a comprehensive discussion of professional liability and risk management, but rather a starting point. For further information on particular matters of interest, residents and others should contact their local, state, and national medical societies, state and federal governments and regulatory agencies, professional associations, or legal counsel. For the American College of Obstetricians and Gynecologists' (ACOG) documents referenced throughout this document, single copies may be requested through the ACOG Resource Center via e-mail (resources@acog.org) or by telephone at (202) 863-2518.

In addition to all the hard work and effort of the Committee on Professional Liability and the staff of the Department of Professional Liability/Risk Management in reviewing, revising, and writing this resource, we also wish to thank Penny Rutledge, JD, General Counsel, Vice President of Legal Affairs, and Susannah Frazier, JD, Staff Attorney, Legal Division, for their invaluable contributions.

Willette L. LeHew, MD, FACOG
Chair, Committee on Professional Liability

Albert L. Strunk, JD, MD, FACOG
Vice President, Fellowship Activities
The American College of Obstetricians and Gynecologists

CHAPTER 1

The Elements of Professional Liability

Duty

Breach of Duty

Causation

Damages

It is vital for physicians to have a basic understanding of the legal concepts of professional liability. Unfortunately, such knowledge will not guarantee a career free of professional liability claims, particularly in the high-risk specialty of obstetrics and gynecology. It may, however, decrease the possibility that a claim will be made or increase the chance of successfully defending a claim.

Professional liability is professional negligence. Negligence also is a legal cause of action involving the failure to exercise the degree of diligence and care that a reasonable and ordinarily prudent person would exercise under the same or similar circumstances.

Although physicians can be sued under other legal concepts, such as breach of contract, the negligence action is the primary means used to impose liability on physicians. A professional liability lawsuit is a civil action filed by a patient against a physician, wherein the patient asks for money for any physical, financial, and mental injury allegedly caused by the physician's negligence.

For a patient to successfully sue a physician for medical negligence, four elements must be alleged and proven in a court of law: 1) duty, 2) breach of duty, 3) causation, and 4) damages. All of these elements must be proven by a patient to prevail against a physician in court. Keep in mind that legal proof is different from scientific proof. The law requires proof of these elements by a preponderance of the evidence, which means more likely than not—or 51% likely on a scale of 100%.

Duty

The duty that a physician owes a patient is based on the physician–patient relationship. A physician's obligation to a patient begins when the physician offers to treat the patient and the patient accepts the physician's services. Residents, however, usually do not have the freedom to pick and choose their patients. Once treatment has begun, the physician has an established duty to the patient and is obligated to follow through with the relationship. Generally, a physician may refuse to establish a physician–patient relationship with an individual. One exception is a patient who appears at the emergency room for care. In this situation, a resident or physician-member of the faculty's attending staff does not have the option to refuse to treat a patient. In addition, federal law restricts the transfer of patients with emergency medical conditions, including women in active labor, in all hospitals that receive Medicare funding (see chapter 12 for more information).

In general, a physician's duty to a patient is to provide the degree of care ordinarily exercised by physicians practicing in the same medical specialty. Residents were once held to an average or reasonable resident standard, which required that a resident possess such skill and use such care as other medical school graduates in residency training. This is no longer true; typically, residents are held to the same standard as fully trained specialists. Therefore, a resident in obstetrics and gynecology is held to the same national standard of care as a board-certified obstetrician–gynecologist.

An Indiana case illustrates this shift in resident responsibility. In this case, two first-year residents were sued for medical professional liability. They allegedly administered lithium during a 2-day period to a patient who showed signs of lithium poisoning. As a result, the patient suffered severe neurologic damage. The two residents, one in psychiatry and one in obstetrics and gynecology, held only temporary medical permits and were "not yet eligible for an unlimited license to practice medicine."

On the issue of what constituted the appropriate standard of care, the trial court held that the residents were required to exercise the same degree of care as other first-year residents under similar circumstances. The plaintiff appealed this decision and the Court of Appeals of Indiana reversed it. The Court of Appeals reasoned that, although the residents were not "physicians" for the purposes of Indiana law, as practitioners of medicine, they were "…required to exercise the same standard of skill as a physician with an unlimited license to practice medicine." The court also emphasized that the residents "…made no representation to the [plaintiffs] that they possessed less skill or knowledge than that normally possessed by practitioners of medicine, and the [plaintiffs] were entitled to rely on their representations that they were doctors as admissions they would be held to the standards of any other practitioner of medicine." *Centnan v. Cobb*, 581 N.E. 2d 1286 (Ind. App. 1 Dist 1991).

A physician owes the patient a duty to practice in accordance with the standard of care. It is difficult, however, to define exactly what is meant by the standard of care. Generally, the standard of care or duty owed to a patient functions as a measurement of the actions of physicians sued for medical professional liability. Hospital protocols and national specialty guidelines frequently are used to establish a standard of care. In theory, the law designates a uniform standard by which juries or judges determine whether a physician has breached a duty to a patient. In practice, however, the standard of care is not a uniform measure and it is imposed on physicians on a case-by-case basis. It most often is established by an expert witness, and the court or jury determines what weight to give to the expert's testimony.

This point is exemplified by a North Carolina professional liability case involving a complication of a cesarean delivery. An obstetrician–gynecologist cut an infant's cheek while making an incision for a cesarean delivery, resulting in a scar of approximately 2 cm. He "admitted he cut the cheek, but denied any negligence, asserting such a laceration is a normal risk of a caesarean section procedure." He further indicated that the procedure was complicated "by several factors, including the muscle of the uterus was thinner than usual, the baby had little amniotic fluid present due to a lengthy period of labor, and there was not any good landmark for the difference between... [the baby's head and the muscle of the mother's uterus]...." Conversely, the plaintiff's expert testified that "...the proper standard of care required...[the physician]...to exercise sufficient care...to not cut the baby." The jury awarded the child $18,000 in damages and the physician appealed.

The appeal was based on the argument that the plaintiff submitted insufficient evidence to meet the burden of proof as to the physician's negligence. Thus, the case should have been dismissed and should not have been sent to the jury. The Supreme Court of South Carolina concluded differently. It stated that the "expert's testimony was evidence that [the physician's] action deviated from the recognized and generally accepted caesarean procedure" and it was proper to send the case to the jury for deliberation. *Bowie v. Hearn*, 292 S.C. 223; 355 S.E. 2d 550 (S.C. App. 1987); 364 S.E. 2d 469 (S.C. 1988).

Breach of Duty

Breach of duty occurs when a physician fails to meet the standard of care in treating a patient. For specialists, such as obstetrician–gynecologists, the standard is defined as that level of skill exercised by physicians practicing the specialty. A plaintiff must show that either an act of commission, "doing that which should not have been done," or an act of omission, "not doing that which should have been done," took place.

Courts rarely distinguish between duty and breach of duty in professional liability cases. Because a physician–patient relationship usually exists, the courts usually focus on breach of duty (ie, deviation from the standard of care). For the plaintiff to prevail, however, duty and breach of duty must be established as separate elements. As noted previously, expert witness testimony usually is required to establish the appropriate standard of care and whether a violation of the standard occurred (1).

Causation

Causation is the most difficult element to prove in a lawsuit for negligence. A patient cannot recover damages unless he or she can prove that the breach of the physician's duty—the violation of the standard of care—directly caused the patient's injuries.

Expert testimony usually is essential to proving the existence of the element of causation. A plaintiff's expert witness must be able to state that the violation of the standard of care caused the patient's injuries to a reasonable degree of medical probability. In legal terms, medical probability means that the injury was "more likely than not" caused by the physician's breach of the standard of care.

Damages

Damages are the final element that must be proven to sustain a medical professional liability cause of action. Damages in a medical liability case are defined as the sum of money a court or jury awards as compensation to a patient for an injury that has been proved to be caused by a physician's negligence. To recover damages, it must be established that the plaintiff suffered physical, financial, or emotional injury caused by a physician's violation of the standard of care.

Damages include compensation for a wide range of injuries that the law has identified and classified into specific categories. The more common categories include special damages, general damages, and punitive or exemplary damages. The courts do not always adhere strictly to these categories, because they can overlap and vary from jurisdiction to jurisdiction.

Special damages are awarded to a plaintiff–patient for expenses that are directly related to, and are an actual consequence of, the injury suffered. Examples of special damages are a plaintiff's out-of-pocket losses, such as medical expenses, lost wages, and the cost of rehabilitation.

General damages are those that the law presumes to accumulate from the natural consequence of the negligent act. A plaintiff can be compensated for both physical pain and emotional suffering. Courts recognize that mental and emotional distress is just as real as physical pain. General damages, therefore, are intangible damages, such as pain and suffering, disfigurement, and interference with ordinary enjoyment of life.

Punitive or exemplary damages are financial compensation to a plaintiff over and above actual losses or expenses and may be awarded along with special or general damages. Although punitive or exemplary damages are frequently claimed in medical professional liability cases, they are rarely awarded. The purpose of punitive damages is to punish a wrongdoing that is outrageous in character. The act need not be intentional, but it exhibits a reckless disregard for a patient's well-being or incompetent treatment of a patient. Examples of such behavior might include a physician who is under the influence of alcohol or drugs when treating a patient, or one who fails to respond to multiple calls to go to the hospital. (See the glossary for definitions of medical–legal terms.)

CHAPTER 2

The Stages of a Medical Professional Liability Lawsuit—Pretrial Stage

Incident Management

Notice of a Claim

Discovery Procedures
   Interrogatories
   Request for Admission of Facts
   Request for Admission of Genuineness of Documents

Depositions
   Definition
   Preparation for a Deposition
   Conduct at Deposition
   Deposition of Another

Physicians who are sued while still in residency may have little say in the management of a lawsuit. A resident will probably not be assigned a personal defense counsel, but will be required to participate in a joint defense. This defense may include the hospital and other staff physicians who participated in or supervised the patient's care. Because of this, residents may find that the attorneys representing them are not "their" attorneys, fully representing their specific interests. Chances are residents will not be a party to defense tactics and strategy. Residents also may be informed of decisions affecting the defense of the case after the decisions have been made.

Physicians who have finished residency and are being sued for incidents that occurred during residency may have more influence over the situation. At this stage, physicians will be in stronger bargaining positions because their standing as residents is no longer being evaluated. Physicians may have more time and financial resources to protect their interests and "rock the boat," if necessary.

No matter when physicians are sued, there may be times when it is appropriate for physicians to consider hiring personal attorneys to protect their interests as opposed to attorneys assigned by the insurance carriers. The two most frequent reasons for employing personal counsel are 1) a conflict of interest on the part of assigned counsel and 2) an exposure to a monetary award that is in excess of the limits of the institutional or personal medical liability insurance policy.

The information and advice found in this chapter applies to medical professional liability lawsuits filed during and after residency. This chapter also provides additional recommendations for physicians participating in their defense after completion of their residencies.

Incident Management

An incident is any event that suggests the possibility of a medical professional liability lawsuit. Appropriate management of an incident is of the utmost importance. Early reporting enables a hospital to act swiftly to initiate loss control measures. Any delay in reporting a suspected problem only compounds the difficulty of preparing a successful defense. As time passes, the ability to complete a thorough investigation becomes increasingly difficult as memories fade, facts become distorted, and witnesses disappear.

A physician's first reactions to an incident can be critical to the outcome of a potential or actual lawsuit. Physicians should follow the procedures established by the hospital for incident management. In most cases, physicians are required to report all incidents to the hospital risk manager. Early notification will allow for a prompt evaluation of the facts, which may strengthen the defense. The risk manager also may give advice on how to best respond to the situation.

There are some signs that indicate that a lawsuit may be coming. These signs include an unanticipated bad result or complication, a direct or indirect expression of dissatisfaction by a patient or a member of her family, failure of a patient to keep scheduled follow-up visits, or requests from an attorney or patient for medical records.

Notice of a Claim

A lawsuit technically begins when the plaintiff files a formal *Complaint* or *Declaration*, a legal document consisting of allegations and legal claims of medical professional liability against the defendant. In medical professional liability cases, it is not unusual for *Complaints* to be filed against multiple defendants. In a lawsuit against a resident, a plaintiff will typically name the hospital and supervising physicians in addition to the resident.

After a *Complaint* or *Declaration* has been filed, the court serves the defendant(s) with a *Summons*. The *Summons* usually is attached to the *Complaint* or *Declaration* and requires an *Answer* to all allegations and issues raised by the plaintiff within a prescribed period.

This matter deserves immediate attention. There are stringent penalties for not responding within the specified period. The defense attorney will prepare the *Answer* and must respond to each of the allegations and issues. Failure to file a timely *Answer* may result in a default judgment against the defendant physician. Failure to respond to allegations or issues may be considered an admission of culpability. The physician's role is outlined in the box.

Responding to a Formal Claim— A Litigation Checklist

- If served with a *Summons*, physicians should stay calm. The first reaction to a *Summons* may be surprise, anger, panic, and self-doubt. Physicians should not overreact or be hostile, but keep their wits about them.
- Physicians should immediately notify the insurance company so that they and the attorney assigned to the case can respond appropriately to the *Complaint* or *Declaration*. Residents usually are insured for medical liability through the hospital's residency program. If the hospital is self-insured, the resident should notify the hospital's risk manager, administrator, or attorney. If the residency program is insured through a commercial liability insurance carrier, the resident should notify the carrier and risk manager or administrator. If it is not clear who should be contacted, the resident should check with the attorney for the hospital that administers the residency program.
- Physicians should deliver the *Summons* (including the attached *Complaint* or *Declaration*) to the hospital's attorney, the assigned defense attorney, and the insurance carrier and retain a photocopy. Physicians in private practice should deliver the *Summons* to their insurance carrier.
- The defense attorney will prepare a written *Answer* to be filed within the period prescribed by the *Summons*. The attorney must respond to each allegation in the *Complaint* or *Declaration*. Physicians may or may not be asked to assist the attorney in preparing the *Answer*.
- The assigned defense attorney will probably ask the most senior physician who was involved in the patient's care to prepare a thorough analysis of the case. This might include a detailed evaluation of all medical records, correspondence, X-rays, and laboratory tests.
- The attending physician, supervising physicians, or residency program director, as appropriate, also will educate the defense team on the medical facts involved in the case. If a resident is involved, the analysis will probably include an opinion on the strengths and weaknesses of the case and the quality of care provided by the resident. Residents may be given little opportunity to present their

(continued)

> **RESPONDING TO A FORMAL CLAIM—
> A LITIGATION CHECKLIST** *(continued)*
>
> side of the story and might not be involved in this analysis. When physicians are sued after residency, they may be able to be more forceful in asserting an opinion as to the management of the patient's care.
>
> - A physician may be asked to write or dictate a chronologic history of the patient's treatment and everything known about the case and give it to the attorney. This material will be considered part of the attorney's work product. Such materials, used by the attorney in preparation for litigation, are not subject to discovery by the plaintiff's counsel.
> - Physicians should keep all personal information about the lawsuit, such as copies of correspondence or documents, in a secure and separate file. This will protect the information from being discoverable by the plaintiff's attorney.
> - Physicians must not casually discuss the patient–plaintiff's medical treatment that formed the basis of the litigation with anyone except the defense attorney or appropriate medical consultants.
> - Physicians should not alter medical records in any way. Evidence of tampering with medical records can lead to a loss of credibility in court as well as a substantial increase in the size of an award. Most legal authorities agree that tampered medical records render a case indefensible. Sophisticated scientific techniques are now available to prove alterations or tampering.
> - Physicians should cooperate with the defense team. They should be honest and should not try to hide any facts. An unpleasant surprise is the worst nightmare of a defense attorney.

Discovery Procedures

Discovery refers to pretrial activities that are intended to permit each party to discover information concerning the opponent's case. Discovery also can eliminate unnecessary issues and helps the parties to either settle the case or present it for trial in an efficient manner. Through discovery procedures, attorneys can assess the strengths and weaknesses of both sides. *Interrogatories, Requests for Admission of Facts, Requests for Admission of Genuineness of Documents,* and *Depositions* are four kinds of discovery procedures. *Depositions* are the most important of the discovery procedures; each procedure will be discussed separately.

Interrogatories

Interrogatories are a set of written questions submitted by one party to an opposing party in a lawsuit. The party served with *Interrogatories* must respond in writing, under oath, within a certain period. *Interrogatories* are more important than most people think. Responses made to *Interrogatories* are admissible as evidence at trial; therefore, physicians should make responses that are precise, thorough, and truthful.

Consultation with the defense attorney is essential in drafting the response. Frequently, the scope of the plaintiff's *Interrogatories* is unnecessarily broad and may include questions that have no relevance to the litigation. If this is the case, the defense attorney will help decide which questions need to be answered. Responses to *Interrogatories* may be used to cross-examine witnesses at trial, so they need to be accurate, complete, and truthful. A physician should carefully review all answers before signing them and swearing to their accuracy. The defense team will have to live with these answers throughout the litigation.

Depending on the degree of involvement in the patient's care, the physician may be asked to assist the attorney in preparing *Interrogatories* for the plaintiff to answer. The physician may know critical information about the patient that should be brought out in this format.

Request for Admission of Facts

A *Request for Admission of Facts* is a series of factual statements, usually limited in number, served by one party to a lawsuit on the other party. The recipient is required to admit or deny the factual statements in writing and under oath, within a prescribed period. Once a fact is admitted by the opposing party, that fact is no longer in controversy and can be stipulated to at trial.

A *Request for Admission of Facts* is an important discovery procedure that may be overlooked by some defense attorneys. For example, a physician might be named in a lawsuit for the simple reason that his or her name appears on the patient–plaintiff's medical record. This may occur even if the physician only saw the patient once at 3:00 AM when she requested pain medication. A *Request for Admission of Facts* could be used by the defense attorney to get the physician released from the lawsuit. The defense attorney would have the plaintiff admit to the physician's limited involvement, which probably did nothing to cause the plaintiff's injuries. The attorney could then file a motion to have the physician dismissed from the case. If the physician is the primary defendant in a complicated case, a *Request for Admission of Facts* can simplify the disputed facts and shorten the ultimate trial. In either situation, physicians should ask their attorneys about the advisability of using this discovery procedure.

Request for Admission of Genuineness of Documents

A *Request for Admission of Genuineness of Documents* is a request from one party in a lawsuit to the other. This request asks the opposing party to admit the genuineness of certain documents. In a medical professional liability lawsuit, the documents usually admitted by this procedure would be the medical records. If the plaintiff has had relevant prior or subsequent treatment from another physician or medical facility, this procedure also can be used to admit those medical records without requiring the other physician or the medical records librarian to testify. This procedure is beneficial in simplifying the trial.

Depositions

Depositions are the most important discovery procedure. Each party may examine the other party or any person who may possibly be a witness. The transcript of this examination, officially recorded and taken under oath, is admissible at trial. Testimony at a deposition has great significance; physicians should not be fooled by an informal atmosphere. They should be as prepared for a deposition as for trial testimony. The importance of a deposition cannot be overemphasized—it may be introduced as evidence during the trial.

Definition

A deposition is a question-and-answer session at which the attorneys of both parties are present and involved in the examination and cross-examination of the witness. It has several purposes: to discover facts and supplement testimony and evidence obtained from other sources; to obtain admissions from the opposing party; to lock in the testimony of a witness; to learn the identity of other possible witnesses; to learn the opposing expert's opinions and theories; to narrow facts and issues; and to evaluate the case for settlement.

The procedure at a deposition is different from trial testimony. The plaintiff's attorney will begin the questioning and will be allowed to cross-examine the witness and to ask leading questions. The defense attorney's role will be to object, when appropriate, and instruct the defendant whether to answer the question. After the plaintiff's attorney has completed this questioning, the defense attorney may or may not question the defendant. Physicians should not be surprised or disappointed if the attorney does not do so; in many instances, the attorney is electing to preserve critical defense testimony until the trial.

Preparation for a Deposition

The defendant's preparation for testimony at deposition is vital. This testimony can be used as evidence or to impeach the defendant at trial; what is said during a deposition is under oath. Without preparation, physicians may be trapped into saying something they might regret later. Before the deposition, physicians should thoroughly discuss with their attorneys their knowledge of the facts of the case and the subjects on which they may be examined. A physician's involvement in the patient's care may have been minimal, and the attorney may try to limit the questions the plaintiff's attorney asks. Physicians should be sure to devote sufficient time to preparation.

Depending on the physician's involvement in the patient's medical care, the defense attorney may ask the physician to thoroughly review the entire history of the case and to:

- Know the treatment and be familiar with all pertinent medical records, X-rays, test results, and data to refer to this material easily.
- Review the chronologic summary of the incident and literature and any area of the specialty that may be the subject of questioning.
- Understand the alternative treatment options and be prepared to explain and defend the choice made.

A defendant physician should insist on a timely predeposition conference with the defense attorney. The physician should know what will be expected and be prepared for possible tactics of the plaintiff's attorney. The defense attorney should provide guidelines about testifying and review the danger areas and weak points. If necessary, the defense attorney should ask mock questions and critique the physician's answers.

A defendant physician should be aware of the opposing counsel's tactics, such as repetitious or leading questions. These are calculated to implicate other physicians or to put witnesses on the defensive, irritate them, and wear them down. An attorney asking repetitious questions may ask the same question again and again, with slight changes in the wording. The purpose of this tactic is to provoke anger or cause witnesses to lose their tempers or make damaging admissions against themselves or their codefendants. The attorney asking leading questions is trying to get a "yes-or-no" response by beginning a question with "wouldn't you agree, Doctor..." or "is it not true...." Physicians should think for themselves, and not allow the attorney put words in their mouths. Such questions need not be answered with a simple "yes-or-no" response.

Physicians should beware of hypothetical questions. The opposing attorney may ask a defendant to "assume" certain facts and express an opinion based on those facts. The defendant physician may become trapped into being an expert witness for the plaintiff. Before answering, physicians should make sure that the "assumed" facts are consistent with the case and that their opinions are consistent with their defense. If defense counsel has not entered an objection to such questions, physicians should ask for instruction as to whether to respond before answering.

Physicians should beware of being painted into a corner. Physicians should not boast when asked to acknowledge the breadth of their medical reading, because they may be held accountable for its content. In addition, opposing counsel may try to get a physician to define an "absolute standard of care" in the case. Remember, at trial, any admissions made during the deposition may be used against the defendant.

Physicians should be cautious when asked if someone or a particular text is an authority. The response should be that "medicine is an art and not an exact science." Therefore, physicians should not always agree with everything written by any one author or found in any one particular text. They should ask the plaintiff's attorney to specify the particular section of the text or article, review its language, and carefully consider their response. Although defendants are not expected to be more knowledgeable than the typical physician specializing in obstetrics and gynecology, they should be prepared to demonstrate their command of all relevant clinical issues, including medical issues. If defendants feel it is necessary to refresh their knowledge about any clinical or basic science issue, this should be done before the deposition.

Physicians should not be surprised if the plaintiff is present at deposition. A party to a lawsuit has an absolute right to attend all depositions in person.

Conduct at Deposition

Physicians should take the deposition seriously, even if it is conducted in an informal atmosphere. If the defense has a strong case and performs well at the deposition, the plaintiff's side may be convinced that it has no case. Most legal authorities indicate that the strength of the defendant's testimony is the most critical factor in a case. Even if the case proceeds to trial, the deposition is a good way to prepare for it.

Physicians should learn to be effective witnesses. They should listen carefully to the questions, weigh their responses, and think carefully before answering. Before answering a question, they should allow a short pause; this gives their defense attorneys a chance to object to the question, if necessary. If a question is not clear, the physician should ask for it to be repeated and clarified before responding. Physicians should not equivocate or act in a patronizing manner. Physicians should be honest and not hide facts.

In giving testimony, physicians should speak clearly. They should not ramble or volunteer information outside the scope of the question. If physicians do not know an answer, they should say "I don't know." If the defense attorney objects to a question, the physician should not answer it until instructed to do so. Physicians should not go off on tangents defending themselves. The deposition is not the time to unnecessarily reveal the reasoning and arguments to be offered at trial in support and explanation of the care rendered. The defense attorney may create an opportunity to do so during the questioning.

Physicians should make an effort to remain emotionally cool. They should not argue with opposing counsel or show exasperation, boredom, or fatigue; an emotional outburst may be used to discredit a physician at trial. They should not be upset if the attorneys are friends and converse casually or banter with each other. They should not be confused or appear to be confused by the proceedings; it may suggest equal confusion in treating the patient.

Physicians should dress neatly for testimony. They also should be courteous and take care in their manner, appearance, and remarks.

Deposition of Another

Any party to a lawsuit has an absolute right to attend all depositions in person. Residents might not have the time or resources to exercise this right. In addition, a resident's degree of participation in the patient's care may not warrant attending any depositions. Residents should discuss with the defense teams whether to attend depositions and respect the attorneys' wishes.

In general, the presence of a defendant at a deposition may have an effect on the testimony given. Witnesses are more likely to tell the truth if the defendant is present. Testimony at a deposition is subject to all the responsibilities and penalties of testifying in court. In addition, attendance at the deposition of another is informative and can aid in preparing for a deposition. This is particularly true of the depositions of the plaintiff and all related medical personnel and opposing expert witnesses. A defendant physician also may be able to provide assistance to the defense attorney during the examination depending on the physician's expertise and degree of involvement in the patient's care.

Chapter 3

The Stages of a Medical Professional Liability Lawsuit—Trial Stage

Being an Effective Witness at Trial
  Pretrial Preparation
  Testimony at Trial

Trial
  Opening Statements
  Trial Testimony
  Plaintiff's Case
  Defendant's Case
  Plaintiff's Rebuttal
  Closing Arguments (Summation)
  Instructions to the Jury
  The Verdict
  Postverdict Activity

Being an Effective Witness at Trial

Preparation is vital to trial testimony. All the points made in the previous chapter on depositions are even more applicable to trial testimony. This section will focus on those items that pertain specifically to the trial. A judge or jury considers not only substantive testimony but the appearance, professionalism, and demeanor of all witnesses and parties.

Pretrial Preparation

Generally, what is at issue is one's conduct (actions or inactions), not one's mindset. Open and frank communication between the physician and the defense team is critically important. The lawyer should be told the truth about the case. This includes all the facts, both good and bad. With time, physicians should develop confidence in their defense attorneys and be willing to have faith in their abilities and judgments. The importance of trusting counsel and the defense team should not be underestimated.

The amount of pretrial preparation that will be necessary will depend on the degree of involvement in the case. The more involved a physician is in the case, the more preparation will be required. At the very least, physicians should review the transcript of their depositions and the transcripts of the experts' depositions and understand the strengths and weaknesses of the case.

During preparation for the trial, physicians should not do independent research without approval by the defense team. This does not mean that physicians should not refresh their basic clinical knowledge about relevant issues of the patient's case.

Physicians should ask the defense for practical advice about the trial date. Trial dates are frequently rescheduled, and it will be impossible to block out time away from duties every time a trial date is set. Ask counsel to advise you how to deal with "possible" trial dates as opposed to a firm trial date. Once begun, the trial will claim first priority on a physician's time. It is in the interest of the institution and the residency program to ensure the resident's availability for testimony.

Testimony at Trial

Physicians want juries to focus on medical issues, not their personalities. The following *do's* and *don'ts* should be helpful for physicians during testimony at trial:

- Physicians should tell the truth in an articulate, respectful, and courteous manner. Physicians should not act smug or project an attitude of "I know it all."
- Physicians should speak directly to the members of the jury, never talking down to them. Physicians should avoid overly technical and scientific terms, instead, communicate with and educate the jury in layman's terms as if explaining a procedure to a patient.
- Physicians should be aware of body language, which can send the wrong message to the jury. Slouching may indicate sloppiness. Placing a hand over one's mouth while speaking may indicate something to hide. Folded arms may be considered a defensive gesture.
- Physicians should be aware of nonverbal communication or distracting habits. Scowling, fidgeting, tugging an ear, hand-wringing, or fingernail biting can send inaccurate signals to the jury.
- Physicians should be aware of how to dress—be neat and simple, not ostentatious.
- Physicians should be aware of speech mannerisms. They should not fill their testimony with "umms" and "you knows," mumble, or speak too rapidly.
- Physicians should not panic if caught in a testimonial misstatement. The defense attorney will present an opportunity on redirect examination to explain inconsistent responses.
- Physicians should not accept the opposing counsel's summary of their testimony unless it is accurate.
- Physicians should not guess at an answer.
- Physicians should not volunteer more information than the question asks.
- Physicians should not be surprised if the judge asks a question; answer it unless the defense attorney objects.

- Physicians should not lose their tempers; they should remain calm.
- Physicians should not manifest relief, triumph, or defeat when leaving the witness stand. It is best to walk with confidence at a normal pace.

Trial

In preparing for trial, physicians should follow the same steps as for preparing for deposition. It is vital that physicians become very familiar with the transcript of their depositions. Physicians need to prepare mentally to hear criticism about their conduct (actions or omissions) during the presentation of the plaintiff's case. Physicians should be aware that during the plaintiff's case every witness and every piece of evidence is intended to show the defendant's conduct in the worst light possible. This can be very difficult to experience. This is the stage of the trial where it is the easiest for defendants to second guess themselves, lose confidence, and lose hope of winning the case. One can be overcome by a feeling of despair. Physicians must realize that the defense team will have its opportunity to build a defense during the defendant's case in exactly the same manner by producing supporting witnesses and evidence that will show the physician's conduct in the very best light possible.

Jury selection takes place immediately before the trial begins. The defense attorney might want the physician to participate in this activity. A typical trial consists of opening statements, trial testimony, closing arguments (or summation), instructions to the jury, the verdict, and postverdict activities.

Opening Statements

The purpose of the opening statements is to allow the attorneys to tell the jury what they intend to prove or what the evidence will show. The plaintiff's attorney goes first, because the plaintiff has the burden of proof. The defense attorney may follow or may wait to give the opening statement until the beginning of the defendant's case.

Trial Testimony

The facts of the case are presented to the jury through various witnesses and exhibits. Evidence is brought forth in an effort to ascertain the truth and to resolve disputes between the parties.

The testimony of witnesses is obtained by direct examination and cross-examination. Direct examination is the questioning of a witness by the attorney who has called that witness to the stand. The attorney may not ask leading questions during the direct examination of a witness. The only exception is the "hostile witness" rule. A hostile witness is a witness whose sympathies are with the other side, but who is believed to have information that might be helpful to the party calling the witness. If the judge determines that a witness is hostile, the attorney is allowed to cross-examine the witness. For example, if a defendant physician is called by the plaintiff's attorney, he or she will probably be declared a hostile witness and be subjected to leading questions. Remember that the plaintiff's attorney may call the defendant physician as a witness on the plaintiff's case. This could mean that the defendant physician is called to testify as the very first witness for the plaintiff, immediately after the opening statements. If the plaintiff's counsel knows or is reasonably confident that the defendant will be in court for the opening statements, counsel may not serve a subpoena on the defendant before the trial to preserve the element of surprise. Physicians must be aware of this possibility so they will not be caught unaware or unprepared. Cross-examination usually is the subsequent examination of a witness by the opposing attorney who may ask leading questions during cross-examination.

Plaintiff's Case

The goals of the plaintiff's attorney are to establish for the jury that the defendant was negligent (breached the standard of care) and that the negligence caused the plaintiff's injury (causation). The plaintiff has the burden of proving these goals by a preponderance of evidence. The plaintiff attempts to meet this burden by introducing evidence through witnesses, medical documents, and exhibits. Because of the medical knowledge physicians possess, they can be instrumental in helping the defense team with cross-examination of the opposing expert witness. If the plaintiff has not introduced sufficient evidence, the defense may request and be granted a directed verdict. A directed verdict ends the trial, although appeals may be requested from directed verdicts (directed by the judge) as well as jury verdicts.

Defendant's Case

The goals of the defense attorney are to prove there was no negligence or the plaintiff's injuries were not the direct result of the defendant's negligence. The defendant's attorney will attempt to meet these goals by introducing evidence through medical documents, witnesses, and exhibits. Important evidence for the defense will be the testimony of the involved medical personnel. The jury wants to hear and see them testify so they can determine the "what and why" of their conduct and how they hold up under cross-examination by the plaintiff's attorney. The key is for them not to be too anxious to tell their side of the story to the jury. Physicians should be patient and work with their attorneys so the jury can hear and understand the case.

Plaintiff's Rebuttal

After the defense has rested, the plaintiff has the right to rebut any new evidence that was introduced during the defendant's case. The law gives the plaintiff the right to rebut testimony because the plaintiff has the burden of proof.

Closing Arguments (Summation)

The attorneys' final arguments to the jury are presented in the closing arguments, or summation. They may, but are not required to, summarize their cases and argue why their clients should prevail. In most jurisdictions, the plaintiff's attorney goes first, followed by the defense attorney. The plaintiff's attorney is given a final opportunity to argue after the defense attorney's summation.

Instructions to the Jury

The judge instructs the jurors on the applicable law for the case. The judge explains through these instructions the legal principles that apply to the case and provides guidelines for the jury's deliberations. The judge also will read a damages instruction. Jurors are told not to consider damages unless they first find for the plaintiff on the issue of medical professional liability.

The Verdict

The verdict is the formal decision or finding made by a jury or judge. The verdict must be in favor of either the plaintiff or the defendant. Verdicts may be split, however. For instance, the jury may find that the hospital's actions were negligent but that there was no negligence by the resident or the supervising physician. Damages are awarded against the responsible party when the verdict is in favor of the plaintiff. In some states, the jury may be asked to apportion fault by percentage among the defendants, which often controls how the judgment is paid.

Postverdict Activity

A case is not necessarily finished once the jury issues a verdict. The losing party has several options:

- Ask the trial court to set aside the verdict and grant a new trial
- Ask the trial court to change the verdict by entering a judgment in favor of the losing party
- Ask the trial court to decrease the amount of the damage award
- Reopen settlement negotiations, using the threat of an appeal as leverage
- File an appeal

CHAPTER 4

The Stages of a Medical Professional Liability Lawsuit—Settlement Stage

Mediation

Factors Influencing the Decision to Settle

Settlement of an Incident

Settlement of a Formal Claim or Lawsuit

Whether to settle will be an issue from the time an incident occurs through a final verdict, and perhaps beyond. Although settlement usually is not a formal part of pretrial or trial procedures, many more cases are settled than are tried to a conclusion in court. Physicians should be aware of what a settlement is, when it can be used, and what their rights are.

A settlement is an agreement made between parties to an incident, claim, or lawsuit that resolves their legal dispute. It is a financial disposition of a case without a decision on the merits of the case. In most instances, a payment is made to the plaintiff in exchange for a release. This legal document absolves the defendant from all past, present, and future liability in connection with the incident. Most releases specifically state that the settlement by the defendant is not an admission of fault.

Substantial costs and risks are involved in litigating a case to a conclusion. The longer a case lasts, the more time, effort, and money is expended. Each participant in the litigation process has reasons for preferring settlement (see box).

Mediation

Parties may be ordered to mediate in good faith. This means that there must be meaningful participation by both sides.

The purpose of mediation is to allow parties and their lawyers, at an earlier stage of litigation, to hear the other side's version and viewpoint of the case. It also gives an objective outside party, the mediator, the opportunity to give a nonbiased assessment of the merit of the case. The court or, in some cases, the parties choose the mediator. In mediation, nothing is binding unless the parties agree. In most jurisdictions, the opposing side cannot use anything discovered during mediation if mediation is unsuccessful. Physicians should know the applicable rule of evidence in their jurisdictions before engaging in mediation.

Mediation gives the parties a more realistic appraisal of the case and, at times, brings forward viewpoints not previously considered. Thus, mediation can be a valuable tool to resolve a case. It can save money and time and expedite settlement by getting parties together face-to-face.

ISSUES OF SETTLEMENT

- Judge
  - —Clears the calendar and disposes of cases quickly
  - —May require the parties to participate in a pretrial settlement conference
  - —Can require mediation
- Insurance carrier
  - —Limits defense costs
  - —Establishes a fixed sum for payment
  - —Avoids an uncertain jury verdict
- Plaintiff's attorney
  - —Considers favorable settlement a victory
  - —Ensures compensation for the client
  - —Ensures compensation to plaintiff's attorney for time and effort
  - —Avoids an uncertain jury verdict
- Plaintiff
  - —Ensures compensation for damages
  - —Avoids further delay
- Defense attorney
  - —Avoids an uncertain jury verdict
- Defendant physician
  - —Avoids an uncertain jury verdict
  - —Eliminates further commitment of time and energy to the litigation process
  - —May decrease stress on physician and family
  - —Avoids negative publicity
- Hospital
  - —Avoids negative publicity

Factors Influencing the Decision to Settle

Many factors can influence any discussion of settlement. These factors include:

- Evidence
  - Analysis of the medical care provided
  - Analysis of the standard of care
  - Missing medical records or unavailable witnesses
  - Illegible or altered records
- Expert witnesses
  - Lack of expert support for the plaintiff or the defendant
  - Quality of expert opinion for the plaintiff or the defendant
- Previous decision of a review committee or panel, if any, and whether that decision is admissible in evidence at trial
- Amount of damage the plaintiff has sustained
  - Seriousness of injuries
  - Influence of the "sympathy factor" on a jury
- Verdict potential exceeds the limits of insurance coverage
- Personal defense counsel retained to protect a defendant physician's assets who will demand settlement within the policy limits
- Dollar amount needed to reach a settlement agreement
- Jurisdiction in which the case will be tried
  - Previous jury verdicts in similar cases
  - Length of time needed to litigate the case to a conclusion
- Personality factors
  - Attitude of the defendant physicians: some may be adamant about going to trial; some may not want to invest further time and energy
  - Adversarial attitude or position of codefendants
  - Strengths or weaknesses of individual witnesses
  - Skill and reputation of the respective attorneys
  - Judge's reputation

The possibility of a settlement may be discussed at any time. A case may even be settled at the incident stage. This process often is referred to as aggressive incident management. The mechanics of this type of settlement differ from the mechanics of settlement of a formal claim.

Settlement of an Incident

In the settlement of an incident, the physician or hospital plays a primary role. The insurance carrier is notified. The hospital risk manager or incident manager also is notified if the incident occurred in the hospital. Settlement depends, in large part, on the response of the insurance carrier or the hospital or both. Further treatment of the patient at no cost may be suggested in exchange for release. Some compensation to the patient also may be suggested.

Settlement of a Formal Claim or Lawsuit

In the settlement of a formal claim or lawsuit, attorneys play a primary role. The plaintiff's attorney typically makes a monetary demand for settlement to the defense attorney. The defense attorney responds with denial, acceptance, or counteroffer. If a counteroffer is made, negotiations may continue until the parties arrive at an acceptable settlement figure. Demands or counteroffers can be made at any time, even if settlement negotiations have previously broken down.

The insurance carrier plays a critical role. Authority is retained to negotiate all settlements. The defense attorney may only accept a settlement demand or make a counteroffer with the consent of the insurance carrier or the defendant or both.

The defendant resident's role depends on the rights contained in the contract with the residency program or the resident liability insurance policy. In most, if not all, residency programs, the hospital and defense attorney can agree to settle a medical professional liability case without the resident's consent. Residents will have no right to reject a settlement they think is unjust or accept one they think is fair. However, they may be consulted about their feelings about a settlement. They should ask the defense attorney for information on all settlement demands and counteroffers. Physicians also should be informed of all choices, the risks with each approach, and the alternatives that are available. It is important to remember that all payments for a medical professional liability claim on behalf of a physician, including a resident, in settlement of a claim must be reported to the National Practitioner Data Bank (see chapter 13 for more information on the data bank).

A New York case illustrates a resident's lack of control in the settlement of a medical professional liability case. An orthopedic resident was sued when one of his patients died of respiratory failure following surgery for scoliosis. The hospital's insurance carrier and its attorneys decided to settle the case on behalf of the resident and the hospital for $350,000.

The resident then sued the hospital alleging that the hospital had no authority to settle the case without his authorization and as a result it violated his right of due process. He argued "...that the absence of a 'waiver of consent' clause in his...employment contract mandates that no settlement can be consented to..." if he objects to the settlement. The hospital contended that absent a "...contractual provision giving...the right to object to settlement..." the resident had no such right. Furthermore, the hospital explained "...without contradiction that the custom and practice in the industry is that residents have no right to withhold consent to a settlement within policy limits when they accept the benefit of the carrier's defense and indemnification."

The Supreme Court of New York agreed with the hospital's arguments. It determined that the industry's custom and practice should be relied on when interpreting contracts and denied the resident's "...request to incorporate a legal right into a contract that is silent on the subject." *Melendez v. Hospital for Joint Diseases*, 575 N.Y.S. 2d 636 (N.Y. Sup. Ct. 1991).

Physicians may wish to hire their own attorneys to protect their personal interests. Settlement is one area in which personal defense attorneys can play a significant role. They will serve as an intermediary to the defense team on settlement discussions and negotiations and ensure that the interests of the physicians are represented.

Physicians should take advantage of the expertise of the defense team in the area of settlement. At the very least, physicians should be given an estimate of the chances of success at trial. To try an indefensible case that could have been settled would be a waste of time and effort; however, to settle a defensible case may set a bad precedent and may have adverse implications for a physician's future practice and insurability. Physicians should try to be as realistic and as objective during the process as possible.

Chapter 5

Informed Consent

Degree of Disclosure

State Laws on Informed Consent

The Process of Informed Consent

Informed Refusal

Informed Consent Forms

Informed consent is a legal doctrine that requires a physician to obtain consent for treatment rendered, an operation performed, and many diagnostic procedures. Without obtaining informed consent, the physician may be held liable for violating the patient's rights, regardless of whether the treatment was appropriate and rendered with due care. It is inappropriate for a physician to provide medical care to an individual without obtaining the patient's expressed or implied permission for the physician to act. A patient must give permission to be touched by another. Without permission, such contact can constitute an assault, battery, or trespass on the person being touched.

An important element of informed consent "is the patient's capacity to understand the nature of her condition and the benefits and risks of the treatment that is recommended as well as those of the alternative treatments. A patient's capacity to understand depends upon her maturity, state of consciousness, mental acuity, education, cultural background, native language, the opportunity and willingness to ask questions, and the way in which the information is presented" (2).

Informed consent is a process that should help the patient gain enough information to be able to decide on a specific course of treatment. Consent often is equated with the document a patient signs to agree to the recommended procedure or treatment. Although some form of documentation is necessary for purposes of treatment and legal defense, it cannot replace the exchange of information between the physician and the patient that culminates in the patient choosing a diagnostic or therapeutic option. The signed document is intended to record this process. Having the patient sign a consent form and assuming the consent process is complete is not enough. The types of consent forms used are discussed in "Informed Consent Forms."

A case from Hawaii provides a good illustration of a physician's affirmative duty to obtain the patient's consent.

One of the primary issues in the case was whether the patient's "...failure to read the consent form before signing it constituted contributory negligence." The defendant argued that if the plaintiff was found contributorily negligent or was partially responsible, he should be "...denied recovery because his own conduct disentitles him to maintain the action."

The Intermediate Court of Appeals of Hawaii found the defendant's contributory negligence argument to be without merit. It held that the patient has no affirmative duty of inquiry as part of the informed consent process. Furthermore, the court stated: "...a physician may not fulfill his affirmative duty of timely and adequate disclosure by merely having the patient sign a printed informed consent form. A signed consent form is not a substitute for the required disclosure by a physician....If physicians come to believe (often incorrectly) that their obligation to obtain the patient's informed consent can be satisfied by securing a signature—even that of a drowsy, drugged, or confused patient on an abstruse, jargon-ridden, and largely unintelligible preprinted consent form—the law's reliance on written documentation may come to pervert its central purpose in requiring informed consent." *Keotnaka v. Zakaib*, 811 P. 2d 478 (Hawaii App. 1991).

Degree of Disclosure

A key element in obtaining valid consent is that a patient must be adequately informed. The degree of disclosure required for valid consent varies from state to state and it is the physician's responsibility to be aware of applicable consent laws. The American College of Obstetricians and Gynecologists (ACOG) Committee on Professional Liability reported that:

"Almost universally, informed consent laws have been liberalized in recent years from the relatively paternalistic 'professional or reasonable physician' standard to the 'materiality or patient viewpoint' standard. In the 'professional or reasonable physician' standard, a physician must disclose to a patient the risks and benefits that are customarily disclosed by the medical community for that treatment, test, or procedure. In the 'materiality or patient viewpoint' standard, a physician must disclose to the patient the risks and benefits that a reasonable person in the patient's position would want to know in order to make an 'informed' decision" (3).

A few courts have taken the patient viewpoint standard one step further and have created a "subjective patient viewpoint standard." This standard is based on what each patient would want to know about a given procedure—not what a "reasonable patient" would want to know. Jurisdictions that follow either patient viewpoint standard require that more information be provided to patients than in those adhering to the reasonable physician standard. As the perspective for evaluating the level of disclosure of risks and benefits in informed consent has changed, it has become clear that patients are entitled to participate with their physicians in a process of shared decision making about medical procedures or treatments (4).

The Supreme Court of Idaho did an excellent job of explaining what is meant by the "...professional medical standard for disclosure in informed consent cases." At issue in this appeal was the trial court's decision that the physician "...had adequately informed the plaintiff concerning the risks involved in performing a biopsy of her lymph nodes." The plaintiff alleged that the trial court erred in stating that the physician should "...be held to the standard of care of physicians practicing in the 'same or like community....'"

The Supreme Court, although recognizing the "...wide divergence of views as to the general measure of the physician's duty to disclose," agreed with the lower court. It concluded that Idaho's consent statute "...clearly and expressly establishes an objective medical-community standard..." for "...determining whether a patient has been adequately informed prior to giving consent for medical treatment." The court also said "A valid consent must be preceded by the physician disclosing those pertinent facts to the patient so that he or she is sufficiently aware of the need for, the nature of, and the significant risks ordinarily involved in the treatment to be provided in order that the giving or withholding of consent be a reasonably informed decision. The requisite pertinent facts to be disclosed to the patient are those which would be given by a like physician of good standing practicing in the same community." *Sherwood v. Carter,* 805 P. 2d 452 (Idaho 1991).

The Supreme Court of New Jersey, however, took a different view when it addressed the appropriate standard for disclosure. In this case, the patient alleged that she developed lymphedema as a result of undergoing a biopsy of breast tissue and surrounding lymph nodes. She also contended that she was never told that lymphedema was a risk of the procedure, so her consent was uninformed. The trial court instructed the jury that the professional standard was the standard by which informed consent was determined. The jury found in favor of the defendant.

On appeal, the Supreme Court of New Jersey examined only one question: whether the professional standard was the standard to be used by physicians in New Jersey to inform their patients of the risks of a procedure. The court, in its opinion, reviewed both the "professional" and "prudent patient" standards of disclosure. It also acknowledged that in the past it had followed the professional standard. The court reasoned, however, that policy considerations regarding a patient's right of self-determination were so persuasive that the time had come to adopt the prudent patient standard. The court noted that "…a professional standard is totally subject to the whim of the physicians in the particular community. Under this view, a physician is vested with virtually unlimited discretion in establishing the proper scope of disclosure; this is inconsistent with the patient's right of self-determination."

The Supreme Court of New Jersey defined the prudent patient standard as being "…measured by the patient's need, and that need is the information material to the decision. Thus the test for determining whether a particular peril must be divulged is its materiality to the patient's decision: all risks potentially affecting the decision must be unmasked."

The court also said "A risk would be deemed 'material' when a reasonable patient... would be 'likely to attach significance to the risk or cluster of risks' in deciding whether to forego the proposed therapy or to submit to it." The court ordered a new trial consistent with its opinion. *Largey v. Rothman*, 540 A. 2d 504 (N.J. 1988).

State Laws on Informed Consent

In the past two decades, many jurisdictions have enacted informed consent laws. Some of these laws address the appropriate standard for disclosure. Other jurisdictions dictate what must be included on an informed consent form. There is little uniformity among these laws either on the procedures to which they apply or on what patients must be told. Some are very broad based and include a multitude of procedures. Others are narrow in scope and apply to only one or two procedures. The mandates in these laws should be complied with to the letter. Physicians must know what their states require.

The Process of Informed Consent

Even though state requirements vary widely, any informed consent discussion with a patient should, at the very least, cover the following issues:

- The diagnosis and the nature of the condition or illness calling for medical intervention
- The nature and purpose of the treatment or procedure recommended
- The material risks and potential complications associated with the treatment or procedure recommended
- All reasonable alternative treatments or procedures, including the option of taking no action, and a description of material risks and potential complications associated with each option
- The relative probability of success for the treatment or procedure in understandable terms (Physicians should never guarantee a result or suggest a guarantee to patients.)

Sometimes a resident is asked to obtain a patient's consent. If the patient has questions that the resident cannot answer, the resident should consult with the supervising physician for advice.

Consent is "fully informed" only when the patient knows and understands the information necessary to make an informed decision about a treatment or procedure; informed consent is a process, not a form (see box). The notation in the patient's medical record should be as complete as possible. It should include the date the discussion took place, that risks and benefits were fully explained to the patient, the patient had an opportunity to ask questions, and the patient consented to or refused the treatment, test, or procedure. There is no informed consent when the treatment or procedure extends beyond the scope of consent. For example, if the care or the risk associated with the care is substantially different from that contemplated by the patient, the courts may find that the original informed consent was not sufficient.

Special informed consent rules apply in certain circumstances, such as emergencies, situations involving minors, and those rare circumstances where authorization for a treatment or procedure is obtained from a court. In a medical emergency, the physician may treat a patient without obtaining the patient's consent to the treatment or

---

WHAT TO REMEMBER WHEN OBTAINING INFORMED CONSENT

- Include significant others or family members, with permission and as appropriate
- Avoid medical jargon; pay close attention to the patient's literacy level and language proficiency
- Try to make sure there is true understanding by having information repeated back to you
- Allow enough time for questions and answers
- Make notations about high-risk issues discussed (eg, tubal ligation failures, vaginal birth after cesarean delivery risks)
- Remember informed consent also applies to office procedures and to the ordering of prescription drugs
- Answer questions regarding your level of expertise, qualifications, and education honestly

procedure. For a genuine emergency to exist, however, special criteria must be met. The patient must be unconscious or incapacitated and suffering a life-threatening or serious health-threatening condition requiring immediate medical attention. Because the patient is unable to consent in these instances, consent is implied. Implied consent is based on the theory that if the patient were competent, the patient would have consented to the care rendered.

Because emergencies present unique situations, it is particularly important for physicians to document in the patient's medical record the reason the care was rendered. This should include a description of the patient's condition at the time of the emergency, the reason the emergency existed, and an explanation for why immediate medical attention was necessary.

Special informed consent rules apply to minors and raise concerns because the rules vary widely from state to state. Basically, minors are unable to consent to medical treatment, so physicians must obtain consent from a minor's parent or legal guardian when providing all but emergency care. All jurisdictions, however, have enacted statutes modifying this special rule to establish criteria or circumstances under which a minor is permitted to consent to medical care without parental permission.

These statutes usually set a statutory age of consent or relate to the ability of minors to consent to specific types of medical care or both. For example, a statute might permit minors older than 16 years to consent to contraceptive care. It also might allow a pregnant minor to consent to treatment regardless of her age. Most statutes do not deal with all of the issues relating to medical consent of minors; therefore, physicians may have little guidance on how to proceed in some situations. It is important for physicians to know the law in their jurisdictions. As with all patients, a minor should be fully informed before medical treatment is provided.

Informed Refusal

Physicians also may be confronted with situations in which a patient has refused medical treatment necessary to save her life or that of her fetus. These are difficult situations, because they typically involve religious or ethical considerations. In these circumstances, a resident should promptly consult with the supervising physician. Although there is not always a "right" way to proceed in these difficult situations, ACOG's Committee on Ethics makes the following recommendations:

> "Every reasonable effort should be made to protect the fetus, but the pregnant woman's autonomy should be respected.... The role of the obstetrician should be one of an informed educator and counselor, weighing the risks and benefits to both patients as well as realizing that tests, judgments, and decisions are fallible. Consultation with others, including an institutional ethics committee, should be sought when appropriate to aid the pregnant woman and obstetrician in making decisions. The use of the courts to resolve these conflicts is warranted only in extraordinary circumstances" (5).

When the medical treatment is refused, the refusal should be documented in the patient's medical record. If the refusal for medical treatment is truly informed and the refusal is documented, physicians should be protected in the event of a medical professional liability lawsuit stemming from the consequences of the refusal (3).

Informed Consent Forms

Informed consent is a process, not a form. One aspect of this process involves obtaining documentary evidence of a patient's consent to treatment. Physicians will be asked on many occasions to obtain this evidence by using a printed consent form. In some states, a signed consent form creates a rebuttable presumption of a valid informed consent on the part of the patient. In states without this type of legislation, a consent form is but one piece of evidence for the defense in a case alleging lack of informed consent.

There are three basic ways in which consent may be documented. The use of one form of documentation instead of another depends on the requirements of state law, as well as institutional policy. The traditional long form usually is very detailed and contains all pertinent information regarding risks, benefits, and reasonable alternatives to a particular treatment or procedure. This form usually includes space to insert special information relevant to the needs of a particular patient.

The second type of documentation is the short form. This form differs from the traditional long form in that it does not contain many specific details; it merely indicates that the risks and benefits of the treatment or procedure have been explained to the patient. Both the traditional long form and the short form usually are used at the institutional level and are signed by the patient or her representative.

The third type of documentation is not a consent form at all; instead, it involves writing detailed notes in the patient's medical record. All information disclosed to the patient is documented, including details regarding risks, benefits, and reasonable alternatives. Any questions asked by the patient and the answers given might be recorded. If there were any witnesses to the consent process, their names also should be included in the medical record. In any event, it should be noted in the progress notes that the informed consent process took place.

Often, the first or second type of consent is combined with the third. Some may prefer this "double consent" as additional evidence against informed consent litigation. The third type of documentation should never be used alone to document the consent process when statutes require a signed, written authorization from the patient. Physicians should check hospital procedures to see if one type of consent is preferred. Above all else, physicians should be aware that there must exist some evidence of consent—oral or written, expressed or implied—granting authority for the physician to proceed, or there must exist some evidence of circumstances in which consent could not be obtained (eg, emergency care).

CHAPTER 6

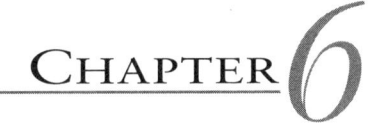

Risk Management Issues

Risk Management in the Hospital Setting
   Communication Between Attending Staff and Residents

Risk Management in the Outpatient/Ambulatory Care Setting

Risk Management in the Hospital Setting

Risk reduction strategies should begin with the first patient–physician interaction. Often that initial encounter takes place in the hospital setting where the resident functions as a member of the health care team under the supervision of an attending physician.

A patient's surprise and disappointment with her treatment may lead to litigation. Therefore, it is vital to convey to a patient the possibility of a complication or change in the expected outcome. For example, the patient who experiences a fever, an infection, or an extended hospital stay after surgery is less likely to sue if she was forewarned about possible complications. Once a complication or untoward event has occurred, she should be informed of her progress on an ongoing basis. In addition, it is necessary to inform a patient of the failure rate associated with operative procedures (eg, sterilization). The patient who suffers a complication (including neonatal complications) requires additional time, attention, and information. Physicians should be alert and caring.

The medical profession has contributed to the public's unrealistic belief that the physician can always provide a cure or a perfect baby. Physicians can help dispel this myth by explaining in a straightforward manner the realities of medical care and technology. Patients should be helped to understand that a perfect outcome cannot be guaranteed. The chance of a poor outcome unrelated to the quality of care is possible in virtually every medical encounter.

The physician must remember that a patient often is under a great deal of stress and may not fully grasp the situation. Consequently, it may be beneficial during the process of informed consent to summarize the information in writing and allow the patient and her family to review and digest all that has been explained. The patient can then ask additional questions to clarify any misunderstandings.

One of the most important methods of communication is the medical record. Examining medical records for clarity and completeness is essential. Reviewing a patient's medical record before she is examined should be automatic. This review should include checking orders and reviewing the notes of nurses, attending staff, faculty, other residents, and medical students. A medical record should not be co-signed and merely assumed to be accurate. It is imperative to read and assess it. If a resident disagrees with the evaluation, this disagreement should be discussed with the supervising physician. Proper observation and evaluation of the medical record will demonstrate that timely and appropriate care has been given.

Technologic advances have improved patient care but also have contributed to the creation of new zones of risk for the specialty, as well as elevated expectations on the part of the patient. Keeping abreast of new techniques and procedures is a fundamental part of practicing good medicine. It often is argued, however, that the very existence of certain technology leads to over utilization and, at times, unnecessary intervention. It is necessary for physicians who use any new advances or technologies to be trained properly and to understand the mechanics of the technology. Equipment must be maintained properly and must operate reliably. Product liability can lead to hospital liability. Hospital policy should allow for a backup and cross-check of every system.

Hospital rules and departmental protocols and procedures exist in almost every hospital and have been established to ensure uniform quality of care. In an effort to increase patient safety, decrease medical errors, and minimize liability risk, all members of the health care team must clearly understand the various federal, state, voluntary organization, and hospital protocols and procedures which focus on patient safety. Failure to comply with these various protocols, and especially hospital policies, may be interpreted as a violation of the standard of care. Therefore, physicians should know, understand, and comply with these policies. With the increasing acceptance of national standards of care for specialists in training, residents should be familiar with national guidelines. Often, however, hospital departmental protocols are more stringent than national guidelines. In such instances, the resident should comply with the hospital's departmental protocols.

Using risk management techniques can substantially protect all caregivers, including the resident, supervising physicians, and the hospital against groundless claims and decrease the potential for patient injury. Diligence in practice and special attention to those areas that carry additional risk will help decrease liability problems. Keeping up-to-date on current literature and technologic advances, maintaining complete records, properly obtaining informed consent, responding to complications in a timely manner, complying with local rules and regulations, and, most importantly, developing effective communication skills are activities that need to be incorporated into everyday practice.

Communication Between Attending Staff and Residents

One of the most common reasons for patient injury and subsequent medical professional liability claims is a breakdown in communications between the members of the team caring for the patient. The "team" includes *all* of the physicians, nurses, and ancillary personnel involved in the patient's care. Communication between attending staff and resident staff is very important. From the attending physician's standpoint, it is obvious that the plan of care must be discussed with the resident. The attending should assure him or herself that the resident understands what is needed (based on the level of training), and the resident should be assured of the attending's availability and willingness to discuss any questions or problems that occur. The attending should communicate any new decisions about the patient so the resident is not surprised by a change in the treatment plan or an additional procedure or test that is ordered without the resident's knowledge. The resident, similarly, should communicate any changes in the status of the patient to the attending. The resident should not feel entirely responsible for the patient's care; a resident is an integral part of the team looking after the patient. There should be a high degree of comfort in calling the attending with concerns or questions about the patient. The issue of whether to report to the attending in the middle of the night could best be answered by the resident's asking, "If I were this patient's attending physician, would I want to know what is happening?" or "What is the worst scenario that could evolve from this situation?" If the resident answers that he or she would want to know, or if the resident is not sure whether the attending physician would want to know, or if there is the potential for significant deterioration of the patient's condition if the worst-case scenario occurred, the resident should make the call. Attending staff would rather learn about a potential problem in the middle of the night than be "blindsided" by a significantly sicker patient when they arrive for rounds in the morning. Even for those patients who are primarily being cared for by residents, staff physicians usually are ultimately responsible for the care given. Thus, the responsible attending should be notified of any change in the patient's status as soon as possible.

In the outpatient setting, the patient's condition should be discussed with the attending physician or preceptor before the patient leaves the unit. In the triage or emergency room, the staff physician should be notified when the initial evaluation is completed so that history, physical examination, and laboratory and imaging studies can be reviewed. A differential diagnosis can then be discussed and a plan of action can be outlined.

If a patient is admitted to the hospital, daily communication is essential. Regardless of the location, the responsible attending physician should be apprised of any complications or unexpected problems at all times.

Risk Management in the Outpatient/Ambulatory Care Setting

In many circumstances, patient care in the outpatient setting will provide residents with the opportunity to familiarize themselves with situations that will mimic those found in a private practitioner's office.

Generally, significant numbers of patients need to be seen in a short period. The outpatient visit often is the first contact the resident has with a patient. Therefore, it is essential that the patient's medical record be reviewed before the initial face-to-face encounter. Residents should pay particular attention to the last several entries. If tests or consultations have been ordered, residents should check to see that the test results and reports have been included. If the test results and reports are not in the medical record, the patient can be asked during the examination whether she has undergone the testing or consultation and where. These results need to be found and reviewed. If she has not, the resident should attempt to determine why and review the importance of why the tests or consultations were ordered.

Physicians should use active listening techniques as well as asking comprehensive questions. The patient should be allowed to completely answer the questions. Physicians should use language appropriate to the patient's level of understanding and obtain interpretive assistance as necessary. They should obtain a thorough history and perform a complete physical examination as appropriate, keeping in mind the patient's need for, and right to, privacy. Physicians should be aware that false charges of sexual misconduct or inappropriate conduct in the examination room, although rare, do occur regardless of physician's gender. These allegations can arise because of a lack of clear patient understanding of certain procedures and technologies, such as vaginal ultrasonography. The ACOG Committee on Ethics suggests that both patients and physicians can benefit from having a chaperone present. "Chaperones can provide reassurance to the patient about the professional context and content of the exam and the intention of the physician and offer witness to the actual events taking place should there be any misunderstanding" (6). Residents should be aware of the institution's and residency program's requirements or guidelines on the use of chaperones.

Eventually, every physician will be confronted with a situation in which a patient has suffered a complication or an iatrogenic injury. Part of the training of an obstetrician–gynecologist is to learn how to deal with this type of situation. This type of occurrence should not be managed without input from the patient's attending physician. Therefore, the attending should *promptly* be called on discovery of an error, a complication, or an iatrogenic injury. The attending and the resident should discuss the issues of disclosure, apology, and plans for additional care. When there is a significant complication, the attending physician *and* the resident should meet with the patient and her family. Documentation should be objective, and there should be no finger-pointing or blame suggested for the event. It should include what was disclosed and what the plans are for dealing with the error or complication. There is no room for guessing, conjecturing, or hypothesizing when documenting significant adverse outcomes.

The following suggestions are helpful for physicians to remember while performing their duties:

- Do not neglect to obtain informed consent before performing those procedures your outpatient or ambulatory care facility has identified as requiring it.
- If your outpatient or ambulatory care facility has established screening and prevention programs, familiarize yourself with the guidelines and follow them as appropriate. Always document recommendations made and patient responses.

- If you answer your pager or receive telephone calls in the outpatient setting, do so from a telephone that affords you the best opportunity of protecting the privacy of all involved.
- Keep your documentation up-to-date, complete, and legible.
- When you are "on-call," are you expected to respond to telephone inquiries from patients seen in the outpatient setting? If so, it is critical that you develop a system that allows you to document calls as received. At the conclusion of your "on-call" duty, you must forward all documentation for inclusion in the patients' medical records.

Chapter 7

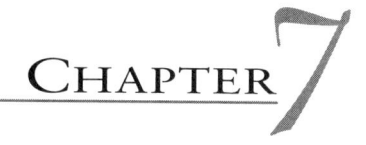

Special Liability Issues for Residents

Liability Status

Ethical Considerations

Liability Status

All residents are trainees under the supervision of others even though some residents are physicians licensed to practice medicine. As employees of residency education programs, residents are under the supervision and control of many different parties during the course of the residency. These parties may include full-time attending staff, volunteer clinical faculty members, more senior residents, the residency program director, and other hospital employees who may have authority over resident physicians.

Even though residents are under supervision, they may be held individually liable for their acts or omissions. In addition, because of the resident's trainee status, those supervising the resident usually are held accountable as well. Generally, liability actions involving residents stem from either the failure to inform patients of a resident's status as a trainee or the failure of a resident to meet the appropriate standard of care. Residents should be identified as residents by their name badges and should explain their status to patients.

A more likely source of liability for residents is the failure to meet the appropriate standard of care. As discussed in chapter 1, residents often are held to the same standard of care as board-certified obstetrician–gynecologists. Residents need to remember, however, that they are not board-certified and that they may not be fully trained in all procedures or treatments. Residents should perform only those procedures or treatments that they are fully trained and authorized to perform. Residents must not have an inflated or unrealistic sense of their abilities. No matter how sincere a resident's efforts to provide all the answers and services to patients, the resident is nevertheless a trainee. No physician, especially a new resident, should expect to be completely knowledgeable in all situations. Courts have little sympathy when physicians, no matter how well intentioned, attempt to perform procedures or treatments that are beyond the scope of their knowledge, training, and experience.

It is the responsibility of both supervising physicians and residents to provide quality care to patients. Communication between residents and supervising physicians is vital in achieving this goal, so both must maintain appropriate continuing communication. This is especially true if residents feel that a patient requires care outside their expertise. Appropriate care must be found, and it is the duty of residents to inform their supervisors of these situations. Communicating the urgency, as well as the scope, of the problem is imperative. In addition, residents should be attentive to the feelings of patients.

In addition to residents' liability for their own negligence, physicians who direct or supervise residents also may be legally responsible for residents' actions. This legal theory is known as vicarious liability. Attending physicians' responsibility for residents' actions arises out of an agency relationship. A person becomes the agent of a second party when that person has been authorized to act for or represent the second party. One form of vicarious liability is known as *respondeat superior* (let the master speak). Under this doctrine, supervising physicians become liable for the negligent acts of their residents. This theory of law also may be extended beyond the clinical faculty member to any physician, such as a private obstetrician–gynecologist, who works with a resident, based on legal concepts such as the "borrowed servant" or the "captain of the ship." Under these doctrines, one party may be liable for the acts of an employee of another if the negligence occurs while the employee is under the first party's direction or control. For example, a surgeon, as captain of the ship, is responsible for the actions of the surgical team whose members are borrowed servants while under the surgeon's supervision. Liability may be imposed even if the surgeon has not aided or encouraged a negligent act. Both the borrowed servant doctrine and the captain-of-the-ship doctrine have different applications and effects in different jurisdictions. Consultation with local counsel is necessary to know whether these doctrines are recognized by a particular state and, if so, to what effect.

In most hospitals and clinics, patients are categorized as a private patient of a supervising physician or a patient of the resident teaching service. The principle of vicarious liability usually applies similarly for both categories of patients. The supervising physician and resident usually are both responsible and liable for all patients for whom they provide care. This holds true regardless of how the patient came under the supervising physician's or resident's care.

A good illustration of the extent to which a court may hold a supervising physician liable for a resident's actions comes from a North Carolina case. The facts in the case are simple. The obstetrician who was responsible for supervising the university's residents in obstetrics and gynecology was providing on-call services from his home 2 miles away from the hospital. The obstetrician began providing on-call services at 5 PM. At approximately 9:45 PM he received a call from a second-year resident in obstetrics and gynecology indicating she had encountered a problem with a delivery. The infant was suffering from shoulder dystocia. The physician left immediately for the hospital. By the time he arrived, however, the infant had already been delivered and "…suffered severe and permanent injuries due to the shoulder dystocia…."

The plaintiff sued the on-call physician alleging that his "…negligent supervision of the residents actually performing the delivery proximately caused the injuries." The supervising obstetrician denied the allegations and argued that "…he owed no duty of care to the plaintiff because no doctor–patient relationship existed." He admitted, however, that he did have responsibility for supervising the residents at the time of the birth. In his defense, the obstetrician presented three affidavits from the heads of departments of obstetrics and gynecology of other teaching institutions in the state in support of his position. The affidavits stated, in part, that a physician could provide on-call coverage "…by either being present in the hospital or, unless a problem is specifically anticipated, by being present at their residence…and immediately available to a telephone…." The plaintiff argued that a supervising physician had a "…responsibility, when he came on call, to find out what obstetric patients had been admitted to the hospital, their condition and to formulate a plan of management." In addition, he argued that the physician should have been aware of the risks of shoulder dystocia in the case because the woman "…was a known gestational diabetic with extreme obesity…." The trial court granted the obstetrician a summary judgment and he was dropped from the case. The plaintiff appealed this decision and the issue was considered by the Supreme Court of North Carolina.

The Supreme Court of North Carolina held that the trial court was incorrect in granting the obstetrician summary judgment. It concluded that the obstetrician "...knew that the residents at the hospital were actually treating patients when he undertook the duty to supervise the residents..." and "...that he owed the patients—including [the injured infant]—a duty of reasonable care in supervising the residents." The court also stated that this duty "...was not diminished by the fact that his relationship with the plaintiffs did not fit traditional notions of the doctor–patient relationship." *Mozingo v. Pitt County Memorial Hospital*, 415 S.E. 2d 341 (N.C. 1992).

Currently, courts in many states are extending the application of the borrowed-servant doctrine and replacing it with a dual-servant doctrine. In this case, not only would a supervising physician be held liable, but the hospital and the residency program also might be held liable for the acts of the resident under the doctrine of *respondeat superior*.

A Missouri case looked at the issue of whether a "...hospital was vicariously liable for negligence of a second-year resident in failing to diagnose testicular cancer." The patient, in this case, "...underwent exploratory surgery of his left scrotum." The resident, under the supervision of a more experienced surgeon, performed the operation. After surgery, the resident informed the patient he did not have cancer. The patient's problems persisted, and 9 months after the first procedure, he had a second operation at the same site. At this time, the surgeon found advanced stages of cancer. The patient died less than a year after the second surgery.

The patient's family brought a wrongful death action against the hospital. The hospital argued that it was not liable for the resident's negligence. The hospital contended that the resident "...was the borrowed servant of the attending surgeon..." and "...the alleged negligence involved the exercise of a physician's medical discretion over which the hospital had no control."

The Missouri Court of Appeals found that the resident "...remained the servant of the hospital during the decedent's operation." This was true, even though the supervising surgeon had "supervisory authority and control" over the resident during the operation. The court also stated that the resident "...was performing the very work for which the hospital had hired and was paying him. In fact, [the resident] was expected to exercise independent medical judgment in the operating room." *Brickner v. Normandy Osteopathic Hospital,* 746 S.W. 2d 108 (Mo. App. 1988).

It is important to remember that a resident may be held liable even though the resident's negligence also can be attributed to another party, such as a hospital or a supervising physician.

Ethical Considerations

The Code of Professional Ethics of ACOG states "If no patient–physician relationship exists, a physician may refuse to provide care, except in emergencies" (7). The moral character of medicine is based on three values central to the healing relationship: 1) patient benefit, 2) patient self-determination, and 3) the ethical integrity of the health care professional (8). In some circumstances, physicians may be asked to provide care that is in opposition to their moral or ethical beliefs.

These ethical considerations give physicians the right to choose their patients. As supervised trainees, however, residents usually do not have the freedom to pick and choose who they will and will not see as patients. Because of this, residents may be asked to render treatment that they consider morally inappropriate (9, 10). When this happens, residents may be confronted with situations that will require making difficult decisions based on what they believe is the right thing to do. These situations may include:

- Being asked to perform a procedure that is beyond their expertise
- Encountering a complication that they are not yet trained to handle while performing a routine procedure

- Being asked to participate in or to perform procedures to which they are morally opposed, such as abortion, sterilization, or in vitro fertilization
- Being confronted with an impaired or incompetent physician who is providing patient care and not being sure of how to proceed

Although this list is not exhaustive, it raises some common moral, ethical, and medical issues residents may have to address.

Before any of these situations arise, residents should determine whether the residency program, the department of obstetrics and gynecology, or the hospital has procedures in place to deal with potential problem situations. Residents also should be familiar with departmental protocols for specific procedures, especially those about which they may feel uneasy, such as abortion. Residents will then know what is expected of them. Furthermore, residents should obtain copies of departmental policies and procedures and the institution's bylaws to become familiar with the proper chain of command within the institution. It also is important to remember that these situations are not new and that, although formal mechanisms to address these issues may not exist in the institution, informal mechanisms might be available.

As trainees, residents should remember that they might not be experienced enough to handle every patient problem. Residents without direct personal supervision should perform only those procedures or treatments that they are trained to perform. Residents may refuse to perform, or ask for assistance with, procedures or treatments that are beyond their skill level. If there are no set procedures in place for a refusal or a request for assistance, residents should follow the appropriate chain of command for the institution. Once these channels are exhausted, it is possible that a substitute or assistance may not be provided. If not providing care would cause the patient more harm, residents should continue to treat the patient to the best of their ability. Residents should then document in the medical record what steps were taken to find substitute or additional care.

Given the ethical questions in everyday medical practice, residents also might confront medical scenarios with moral ramifications. If residents are morally opposed to abortion, for example, they should make that position known to the program director. In this regard, federal regulations applicable to hospitals receiving any federal funding, as well as ACOG policy, hold that no physician should be required to perform an abortion if the physician objects on moral or religious grounds. However, such a position would not preclude caring for a patient experiencing complications of an abortion.

Residents should not wait to object until the first time they are asked to perform an abortion or another procedure that presents a personal moral dilemma. It is best to discuss feelings about such procedures with supervising physicians as early as possible. This gives the supervising physician ample time to make arrangements for substitute physician care. If for any reason the supervising physician refuses a request not to be involved with a procedure, residents should follow the appropriate chain of command to resolve the situation. Residents who elect not to participate in procedures presenting personal moral dilemmas should still be able to counsel patients, make appropriate referrals for alternatives for care (2), and manage post-procedure complications.

Finally, residents might find themselves caring for patients alongside a chemically-impaired or incompetent physician. In this situation, it is always difficult for residents to know exactly what to do or how to proceed. The best advice residents can follow is to use their best judgment, always remembering that patient care is the first priority. Whenever possible, residents should seek the advice of supervising physicians, other physicians associated with the residency program, or the residency's program director. In addition, residents should follow any institutional mechanism available to assist the impaired or incompetent physician in finding help. On occasion, however, emergency circumstances may prevent a resident from consulting with anyone else. If the physician's impairment is causing immediate harm to the patient, a resident may assert authority over the impaired physician and then seek assistance from the senior hospital staff.

Chapter 8

High-Risk Areas for Litigation in Obstetrics and Gynecology

The Neurologically Impaired Infant

Delivery Methods
    Cesarean Delivery
    Vaginal Birth After Cesarean Delivery
    Operative Vaginal Delivery
        Forceps
        Vacuum Assisted Deliveries

Shoulder Dystocia

Breast Cancer

Other Areas of High Risk
    Laparoscopy
    Induction of Labor

There are many areas of high risk for litigation in the practice of obstetrics and gynecology. As science progresses, these areas will change and evolve. Twenty years ago the issues of group B streptococcal infection and whether to allow videotaping of deliveries were virtually nonexistent. Twenty years from now there will be other areas which will become the focus of litigation and claims review.

Obstetrician–gynecologists should be familiar with the types of claims commonly brought against the specialty. Adequate training and education, ongoing patient communication, and thorough documentation remain the clinician's best defense against medical professional liability claims while ensuring safe, high-quality care for all patients.

Even though the overwhelming majority of obstetrician–gynecologists provide excellent care, litigation is an everyday reality for this group of medical specialty physicians. Statistics from the 1999 professional liability survey of ACOG's membership reveal:

- At least 75% of ACOG Fellows have been sued at least once with an average of 2.53 claims experienced during their careers.
- More than one fourth (27.8%) of obstetrician–gynecologists have had at least one claim as a result of care rendered during residency.

The claims data in this chapter comes from *Professional Liability and Its Effects: Report of a 1999 Survey of ACOG's Membership* (11). It is the seventh survey that ACOG has conducted on professional liability issues. Similar to previous surveys, the 1999 professional liability survey provides continuing trend data on liability claims in obstetrics and gynecology. This survey contains data on 1,428 obstetric and gynecologic claims opened or closed during the 3-year period beginning January 1996 and ending December 1998.

The Neurologically Impaired Infant

The most frequent obstetric claims involve neurologically impaired infants and cases of stillbirth and neonatal death. Almost one half (46.9%) of the obstetric claims in the 1999 professional liability survey fit into one of these two categories. Neurologically impaired infant claims accounted for 30.2%, and stillbirth and neonatal death accounted for 16.7% of these claims. There is no question that these types of claims present the most significant liability problems in obstetrics and gynecology. In fact, these statistics have changed very little from 1987 when ACOG first looked at claims in obstetrics and gynecology in detail (12). In the 1987 professional liability survey, which covered any claims ever filed, neurologically impaired infant claims (30.9%) and cases of stillbirth and neonatal death (14.7%) accounted for 45.6% of all obstetric claims.

Neurologically impaired infant claims are expensive. The 1999 professional liability survey reported that the **average** amount paid on behalf of an obstetrician for this type of claim is $935,952 (11). This is more than two and one half as much as the average amount paid for all claims.

Physicians, especially those facing birth-injury lawsuits, should be familiar with the National Institutes of Health report entitled *Prenatal and Perinatal Factors Associated with Brain Disorders* (13) and the body of literature that has followed it.

Delivery Methods

The provision of quality obstetric care often requires physicians to make swift decisions. Residency educational guidelines increasingly recommend that residents act only under the direct supervision of the attending physician or faculty medical staff. However, not all health care institutions can meet that goal. In the absence of an attending or faculty physician, many facilities authorize and direct the fourth-year resident to act in the best interest of the patient, which includes intervening when the safety of the patient or her fetus is in jeopardy.

Whether acting independently or under supervision, residents must continually monitor the progress of labor and ensure the adequacy of the documentation of that process. Antecedent evidence of a potentially difficult delivery often is found in the progress and management of active labor. Before performing any procedure, it is the responsibility of the physician to provide the patient with enough information regarding risks, benefits, and alternatives so she can make an informed decision about whether to proceed. Physicians should consider dictating a procedure note for any delivery, but especially for operative deliveries.

Cesarean Delivery

The 1999 professional liability survey revealed that patients delivered by cesarean delivery accounted for 41% of all obstetric claims, including 50.8% of neurologically impaired infant claims, 46.9% of maternal death, and 45.1% of stillbirth and neonatal death claims (11). However, vaginal deliveries accounted for 50.8% of all obstetric claims, including 43.7% of neurologically impaired infant claims, 43.6% of maternal death, and 52.6% of stillbirth and neonatal death claims.

Vaginal Birth After Cesarean Delivery

According to ACOG's Committee on Practice Bulletins—Obstetrics, a trial of labor following a previous cesarean delivery is an accepted method to decrease the overall cesarean delivery rate under certain circumstances (14). However, physicians must recognize the risks as well as the benefits associated with vaginal birth after cesarean delivery (VBAC). A significant risk is created when patients attempt VBAC in facilities that are not equipped and not staffed to deal immediately with VBAC-related emergencies, such as uterine rupture.

Physicians should become familiar with the criteria that identify candidates for VBAC as well as the contraindications for its use. As with all procedures, the risks and benefits to the patient and her fetus must be thoroughly discussed with the patient and completely documented in the medical record. The 1999 professional liability survey reported that VBAC deliveries were used in 4.6% of the total obstetric claims, in 5% of the neurologically impaired infant obstetric claims, and 17.5% of maternal injury–major claims (11).

Operative Vaginal Delivery

According to ACOG's Committee on Practice Bulletins—Obstetrics, the incidence of operative vaginal delivery (use of forceps or vacuum extraction) is approximately 10–15% in the United States (15). Physicians are advised to become familiar with the relevant clinical indications for its use, possible complications to the patient and her fetus, and the technical skills necessary to perform operative vaginal deliveries.

Forceps

The 1999 professional liability survey reported that the use of forceps was a factor in 10.3% of all obstetric claims (11). They were a factor in 13% of neurologically impaired infant claims, 22.7% of other infant injury–major claims, 13.9% of maternal injury–major claims, and 8.1% of stillbirth and neonatal death claims.

Vacuum Assisted Deliveries

The 1999 professional liability survey reported that the use of a vacuum extractor was a factor in 7.3% of all obstetric claims (11). It was a factor in 11.2% of neurologically impaired infant claims, 17.9% of obstetric informed consent claims, 9% of other infant injury–major, claims, 8% of other infant injury–minor claims, and 8.7% of stillbirth and neonatal death claims.

Shoulder Dystocia

According to ACOG, shoulder dystocia is an obstetric emergency and places the patient and her fetus at risk for injury (16). To minimize the risks to the patient, her fetus, and to the physician, a management plan should be formulated to be used in the event shoulder dystocia is encountered. When confronted with the actual condition, step-by-step documentation of the techniques used, any injury noted, and a description of plans for the infant's follow-up should help decrease the likelihood of future litigation because of the care provided.

The 1999 professional liability survey reported that shoulder dystocia/large baby/large for gestational age was a factor in 17.1% of all obstetric claims (11). It was a factor in 18.4% of neurologically impaired infant claims, 76.4% of other infant injury–major claims, 45.3% of other infant injury–minor claims, and 6.3% of maternal death claims.

Breast Cancer

Failure to diagnose breast cancer continues to be a major liability concern. The SEER Cancer Statistics Review 1973–1998 stated that the lifetime risk for women of having a breast cancer diagnosis is 13.24%

(1 in 7.55) (17). Despite educational efforts aimed at early detection, physicians continue to be sued for failing to diagnose breast cancer. This is documented by data from the professional liability insurance industry and ACOG's 1999 professional liability survey.

The 1999 professional liability survey reported that "failure to diagnose" was one of the most frequent primary allegations (11). Failure to diagnose represented more than one fourth of all gynecologic allegations. If these cases are analyzed further, close to two thirds (63.3%) were cancer related. Of these cancer-related claims, more than one half (53.7%) involved breast cancer. No single other type of cancer came close to equaling this percentage. For instance, failure to diagnose cervical cancer accounted for only 18.1% of these claims.

The Physician Insurers Association of America (PIAA), which represents physician-owned insurance carriers that insure the majority of all physicians in the United States, reported on breast cancer claims in a 1995 study (18). A committee of the PIAA reviewed 487 breast cancer claims that resulted in at least some payment by 33 member companies. One of its findings was that a large majority of plaintiffs who filed breast cancer claims were younger than expected: 60% of plaintiffs were younger than 50 years and 30% were younger than 40 years. The American College of Obstetricians and Gynecologists' 1999 professional liability survey showed findings that are even more striking. It reported on the age of the patient–plaintiff at the time the cancer was diagnosed. More than three fourths of the patients (76.2%) were younger than 50 years when the cancer was diagnosed and more than one half (51.6%) of them were younger than 40 years. The PIAA study recommended that a high index of suspicion for breast cancer in younger women be maintained by treating physicians.

The average amount paid for failure to diagnose breast cancer is costly. According to ACOG's 1999 professional liability survey, the average amount paid, or indemnity, for such a claim was $140,977 (11). The severity of these types of claims should not be surprising because the patients in these types of cases often are young women. Physicians should maintain a high index of suspicion when treating women who report breast pain or have a lump in their breasts, even if the physician is unable to palpate the lump claimed by the patient. Imaging studies or consultative referral should be used liberally.

Other Areas of High Risk

Laparoscopy

The laparoscope has evolved into an important tool in operative gynecology. As laparoscopic surgical procedures become more complex, the number of complications has increased. The 1999 professional liability survey reported that a laparoscopic procedure was a factor in 20.1% of all gynecologic claims, 22.5% of patient death claims, 43.6% of patient injury–major claims, and 34.8% of failure-of-sterilization claims (11).

Furthermore, the PIAA reports that laparoscopic procedures continue to be a condition for which patients frequently file medical professional liability claims. According to the PIAA, between 1991 and 2001, a total of 2,909 claims and lawsuits involving laparoscopic procedures were reported to the Data Sharing System; more than $149 million has been paid in indemnity and more than $40 million has been paid in defense costs of these claims.

Induction of Labor

The induction of labor carries with it benefits and risks, both to the patient and her fetus (19). These considerations must be recognized and addressed. Additionally, physicians should completely document in the medical record their thought processes leading to a decision to induce labor. (For a more thorough discussion of the criteria to be considered, as well as various methods of labor induction, physicians are referred to ACOG Practice Bulletin 10, "Induction of Labor" [19].)

Chapter 9

Patient Communication

Effective medical practice requires a positive interaction between physicians and patients. Communication is a two-way process in which both the physician and the patient have a responsibility to the other. A successful physician–patient relationship depends largely on effective communication skills and the physician's sensitivity to the patient's needs.

Litigation usually is triggered by a bad outcome, but communication problems between physicians and patients can contribute significantly to patient frustration, dissatisfaction, and oftentimes, a lawsuit. Developing good relationships with patients is not only good practice but it also is an excellent way to minimize the chance of lawsuits. It is the responsibility of the physician to establish an atmosphere conducive to communication.

The following 10 steps offer a guide to more effective communication and demonstrate the respective responsibilities of the physician and the patient:

1. Establish a healthy rapport.
2. Respect the patient as a person. Ask how the patient wishes to be addressed.
3. Be honest—be an ally.
4. Obtain an accurate record of symptoms and history.
5. Disclose all relevant facts.
6. Explain clearly any alternatives and reservations.
7. Be sure the patient thoroughly comprehends information, advice, and instructions.
8. Answer all questions.
9. Obtain valid informed consent.
10. Follow-up.

The first three steps concern the human aspects of physician–patient relationships: establishing good rapport, showing respect, and being an ally. They deal with how physicians relate to patients and how a humanistic and professional approach can eliminate problems and decrease negative feelings. It is apparent that some lawsuits are initiated because of the physician's attitude toward the patient, as perceived by the patient.

Physicians should establish a rapport with their patients in the initial contact—first impressions are lasting impressions. They should introduce themselves and describe their role in the patient's care. Patients should not be addressed by their first names unless so requested. Physicians should be neat and well groomed at all times. A disheveled appearance can lead the patient to lose trust in the care she is receiving and worry that her care will be sloppy. Dirty scrubs should not be worn. Physicians should be aware of and understand the fears and anxieties that patients are experiencing and should make patients feel as comfortable as possible.

At this point in physician–patient relationships, the way in which physicians look, speak, and act is as important as what they say. Establish good eye contact—eyes can be a great aid to communication. Physicians should be positive, caring, and respectful. They should remind patients that they are working first and foremost for them.

Physicians should respect patients and understand their beliefs. Patients should be treated as mature, intelligent human beings and dealt with honestly. Physicians should treat their patients as they or a member of their family would want to be treated. Physicians must clearly and honestly explain the nature of their services and make sure that patients thoroughly understand this information. They should communicate in terms patients can understand and avoid being pompous or arrogant.

Physicians should spend the time necessary to answer questions and address any concerns. They should be an ally—honest and open with patients. Residents should disclose their status as physicians who are in training. They should explain the circumstances of the situation, with emphasis on the fact that residents are supervised by more experienced physicians. Patients have the right to refuse treatment by residents. With good communication skills, it is possible to overcome this obstacle and still participate in the care of the woman by outlining the advantages of resident participation.

Steps four through eight ultimately assist in obtaining a valid informed consent, which is step nine. It is the responsibility of patients to describe their history and symptoms honestly and accurately. Frequently, the resident will be the one who will listen to all complaints, diagnose the patient's problems with input from the supervising physician, and recommend treatment or alternatives that appear to promise the best result. It is the patient's responsibility to consider the pros and cons of each recommendation and decide which course of action is best for her. These five steps are all key elements of a valid informed consent process (see chapter 5 for a discussion on the informed consent process). Patients should receive daily updates on their progress. Information from all sources (resident, supervising physician, nursing staff) should be consistent. Inconsistencies, even minor ones may be disconcerting and confusing to patients and lead to apprehension, distrust, and the fear that no one knows what they are doing. This can lead patients to believe that the medical care they are receiving is substandard.

Physicians' responsibilities do not necessarily end immediately after treatment or surgery. Physicians also will probably be responsible for follow-up care (step 10), which may include careful and specific instructions and, if necessary, follow-up visits. Ideally, all instructions to patients should be written in detail and copies should be given to them. A copy also should be placed in the patient's medical record for future reference. Less than optimum outcomes require even greater follow-up.

In summary, effective communication with patients can decrease the risk of medical professional liability lawsuits. Physicians need to remember that good medical care involves treating patients with care, concern, and respect; keeping patients informed; and allowing patients to share responsibility in decision making.

CHAPTER 10

Medical Records

Accuracy

Comprehensiveness

Legibility

Objectivity

Timeliness

Correcting Medical Records

It is important for physicians to have a good rapport with other members of the health care team and to communicate with others at all levels. Lack of communication between members of the health care team may lead to error, which in turn may lead to a lawsuit. The common element in communication among all members of the health care team is consistency in the information given to patients and legible, well-documented medical records.

The medical record is a critical component of good medical care. It chronicles the patient's course of illness and treatment, it provides essential information to all those who subsequently care for the patient, and it is a legal record that helps document that the standard of care was met. A well-documented medical record does not ensure good care. However, a well-documented medical record will allow all practitioners to understand the patient's course. Medical records should be maintained in a professional manner. Moreover, in a courtroom, complete and accurate medical records are the best defense physicians can have. A good medical record suggests that due care was exercised in diagnosis and treatment, while poor medical records (lack of notes, altered statements, erasures, illegible notes) may force the settlement of even defensible claims.

The medical record is a comprehensive database communicating essential instructions and observations. It should provide a permanent, written record of patient care including treatment and the facts and reasoning behind the chosen course of treatment. It is not a place for gratuitous comments or arguments between practitioners.

The importance of good record keeping cannot be overemphasized. Physicians should examine their record-keeping style and habits in light of the following critical elements. If physicians fail to observe these essential considerations in record keeping, they could find those records to be their worst courtroom adversary.

Accuracy

The medical record must be kept current and accurate at all times. Members of the health care team often communicate with each other or with other medical facilities only through entries on a patient's medical record. If the medical records are incomplete, irreparable injuries to patients may occur. The greatest care should be used when choosing descriptive terms, using abbreviations, entering numerals, and recording events. All abbreviations should be uniform and clearly understood by all members of the health care team.

Physicians should be aware of the accepted method of recording entries used by their institution or hospital and adhere to it when making notes in the medical record. When no such policy exists, residents should ask the residency program director for guidance and to recommend an appropriate format for charting. Physicians should be consistent in their use of terminology and selective in choosing terms, such as "extraction" or "delivery," where the careless interchange of terms blurs the accurate interpretation of the actual procedure involved. Abbreviations should not be used unless they are immediately clear to everyone involved (eg, SBE is self breast examination to some and subacute bacterial endocarditis to others). All physicians also should beware of the "wayward decimal"—a tenfold increase or decrease in dosage can be critical and can make a difference between life and death. When calculating dosages of drugs according to body weight, recheck mathematics for accuracy. Confusing drugs with names similar in sound or spelling also can have a serious impact. It is particularly important for medications and their dosage to be written legibly. All events during the course of treatment always should be noted with the time, the date, and a legible signature.

Comprehensiveness

When there are deviations from the standard of care, the rationale and justification should be documented. All notes in the medical record should be dated and timed.

The comprehensive medical record will contain the complete details of the patient's present condition, past medical and surgical history, family and social history, physical examinations, laboratory tests, risk identifications, current medications, and drug reactions. The medical record also will include all visits, progress notes, any consent forms, consultant reports, correspondence, and notes of conversations, whether in person or by telephone. The diagnosis and therapeutic plan should be fully documented in a way that explains the rationale, risks, and alternatives considered. Informed consent should be obtained where appropriate.

The patient's responses to these matters also should be included. Any variance in the patient's compliance with therapy should be noted in the medical record. For instance, a patient's failure to keep appointments should be documented. When a patient refuses to undergo a test or procedure, the informed refusal should be documented in the patient's medical record (see chapter 5 for more information on informed refusal). Notations must be meaningful—record both negative and positive remarks and document all recommendations and essential findings.

It is important to record telephone conversations and to retain copies of telephone messages. A telephone conversation may prove to be crucial in a defense should a serious dispute arise in regard to a particular conversation. It will be difficult for a plaintiff's attorney to convince a jury that the plaintiff's recollection of a conversation was more accurate than the defendant's written notation of that conversation.

Nursing notes also are an important part of the medical record. Physicians should read these notes carefully. Similarly, nursing notes on the fetal monitor strip must be scrutinized. If a physician feels that any entry in the medical record or any other record is incomplete or inaccurate, an annotation should be made about the omitted or erroneous entry. Such corrective entries should not obscure or obliterate the entry in question and should be, whenever possible, strictly factual. As noted hereafter, it is not appropriate to argue or 'joust' in the medical record.

Legibility

Medical records must be legible, clear, and concise. Physicians should remember that medical records are written for others as well as for themselves. Grave consequences can occur when medical records are illegible, making it impossible to evaluate the quality of care or even to determine what care was given. Legibility takes more time but ensures the best possible communication among members of the health care team, especially in critical moments that demand not only accuracy but also an understandable message.

The use of computers to chart notes has alleviated many of the deficiencies associated with hard copy: legibility, date and time of entry, correction of previously entered data. It also has the advantage of allowing physicians to document telephone calls and notes and enter data from almost any computer terminal.

Objectivity

The medical record is not the place to critique or criticize a colleague's work or treatment plan. It is inappropriate to use the medical record for this purpose. If a diagnosis or treatment plan needs to be changed, this can be done according to the current information or a reevaluation of the data without criticizing the preceding care.

One of the major reasons for medical professional liability lawsuits is the failure of physicians to confine their observations in medical records to clinical facts and objective analyses. Unprofessional opinions placed in the medical record endanger the credibility of the record and open the resident, physician, hospital, and the residency program to criticism. Careless talk, open disputes, and second-guessing among colleagues regarding patient care often can lead to unwarranted medical professional liability actions. Loose or unfounded statements should never be made, let alone placed in a medical record. Only facts and clinical judgments are appropriate to include in the medical record. Thus, it is important to avoid casual criticism of the work of other physicians, especially in the absence of facts.

Timeliness

Events should be recorded in the medical record as they occur or become known. Delay only increases the risk of confusion or neglect of important facts and observations. The sequence of events is critical to establishing what information was known and when it was known during the course of treatment. A physician should never delay in dictating or writing an entry in the medical record. In addition, the physician should read and initial all typed entries.

If laboratory tests are ordered, the rationale, as well as the results, should be explained and noted. Laboratory reports should be read and interpreted in a timely manner by the physician and, if necessary, the resident's supervising physician. A mechanism should be in place to ensure that all diagnostic studies ordered or specimens collected are processed, and all test results received and acted on. When electronic fetal monitoring is used for an obstetric patient, all activities should be recorded on the strip and tracings should be retained with the medical record.

Correcting Medical Records

The medical record can be the most important evidence in a medical professional liability trial. Poor record keeping can make it impossible for a judge and jury to determine whether the care was good or bad and can even make good care look bad.

Evidence of tampering with the medical record can lead to a loss of credibility in court and make a defensible case indefensible. It also can substantially increase the size of an award. Moreover, falsely claiming that a record was written without alterations can leave physicians open to a perjury charge. If it is necessary to correct an entry in the medical record, residents should bring it to the attention of their attending physician immediately. The proper procedure for correcting an entry should be used by all physicians (see box). The correct entry should be placed after the last entry, the change explained, and the change dated and initialed. Physicians should not attempt to supplement, complete, or clarify the medical record after notification of a claim. Changes or inconsistencies in the medical record and destroyed or mutilated medical records suggest that it has been altered, which in turn suggests that physicians have something to hide.

Whether operative notes should be dictated on all deliveries may be debated but operative notes should certainly be dictated on all complicated and operative deliveries. This would include forceps and vacuum deliveries and those involving shoulder dystocia.

Do's and Don'ts of Correcting Medical Records

Do
- Single-line through erroneous entry
- Initial
- Time and date new entry

Don't
- Scratch out or "white-out" error
- Write over an entry
- Introduce new material in previously written notes
- Try to squeeze notes in margins or at very bottom of the page

CHAPTER 11

Professional Liability Insurance

Professional Liability Insurance Coverage During Residency
    Insurance Checklist for Residents
    Types of Liability Insurance Coverage
    The Amount of Insurance Coverage
    Restrictions on Liability Insurance Policies for Residents
    Future Considerations for Residents

Professional Liability Insurance Coverage After Residency
    Types of Liability Insurance Coverage
    Exclusions from Liability Insurance Coverage
    Options for Settlement of Claims
    Types of Insurance Carriers
    The Liability Insurance Carrier–Physician Relationship

Professional Liability Insurance Coverage During Residency

Most residents in obstetrics and gynecology have been exposed to the dangers of professional liability lawsuits and are aware of the effect that these lawsuits have on the specialty. But there are hidden professional liability issues for residents that do not have anything to do with lawsuits or risk management, and they can have a significant impact on a resident's future ability to practice medicine. These hidden issues are related to insurance.

Insurance Checklist for Residents

Residents often assume that professional liability insurance is provided for them by their residency programs. A residency program survey on professional liability insurance, conducted by ACOG's Department of Professional Liability/Risk Management, justifies this belief. All of the programs responding to the survey provided some form of professional liability insurance for their residents in obstetrics and gynecology. Knowing that insurance is provided, however, is not enough. Residents also need to know:

- The type of coverage provided by the residency program
- Whether coverage for incidents occurring during residency will be provided if they become claims after a resident leaves the program
- The dollar amount of the insurance coverage and the dollar amount of tail coverage, if applicable
- Any and all limitations on practice contained in the insurance policy
- What effect claims might have on a resident's ability to obtain liability insurance in the future

Residents also should obtain and keep copies of the master professional liability insurance policy for the residency program or a written statement or certificate of the coverage provided. Some residency programs are self-insured. This means the hospital or residency program directly assumes the risk for all medical professional liability claims. Residency programs also can be insured through commercial insurance carriers. Other programs may both be self-insured and have a policy with a commercial carrier for insurance coverage above a certain dollar amount. For example, the hospital or residency program may be self-insured for $3 million but have insurance for any settlement or judgment higher than $3 million.

Types of Liability Insurance Coverage

There are two basic types of professional liability insurance: occurrence coverage and claims-made coverage. Occurrence coverage covers residents for all claims resulting from the period covered by the policy, regardless of when the claim is made. Residents covered by an occurrence policy will be covered for all medical professional liability claims arising from incidents during their residency, even if, as is often the case in obstetrics, a claim for an impaired infant is made years after the residency is completed. Residents should be aware, however, that the policy's liability limits for future claims will be identical to the limits of the policy during residency. For example, if the institution provides $1 million/$3 million coverage and a resident is sued 20 years later for an incident that occurred during residency, these same policy limits will apply. Problems could arise if the amount of the coverage is not sufficient to cover potential settlements or judgments in the lawsuit.

Claims-made insurance covers residents for all claims reported during the period covered by the policy. The insurance company does not have an obligation to cover claims that are made after a policy's expiration date. To protect against later claims, insurance companies provide a special policy called "reporting endorsement coverage." This is popularly known as "tail coverage," although the policies always use the term reporting endorsement coverage. Tail coverage must be purchased when the claims-made policy expires. If it is not purchased, residents will not be insured for any future claims that involve incidents that occurred during residency.

Residents also should be familiar with the tail's liability limits, the period these limits apply, and whether these limits are renewable. Generally, the tail's liability limits will be identical to the claims-made policy's limits. For instance, if the claims-made policy limits are for

$1 million/$3 million, the tail's liability limits will be for the same amount. The period these limits apply, however, varies between insurance carriers. Some insurance carriers apply the stated liability policy limits to the entire period the tail will be in effect. For a $1 million/$3 million tail, this means that the insurance carrier will pay up to $1 million per claim and up to a total of $3 million during the course of the policy. Once the $3 million payout is reached, regardless if this occurs 1 year or 10 years after the purchase of the policy, the physician will be responsible for paying all future damages. Other insurance carriers renew the tail's limits annually until the physician's estate goes through probate. Still other carriers will renew the limits for only 3 or 4 consecutive years after tail coverage is purchased. After the last renewal, the physician will be responsible for all future damages in excess of the tail policy aggregate. Given all the ways tail coverage operates, it is important to investigate the intricacies of how a residency program's tail coverage functions.

In recent years, claims-made coverage has become more popular than occurrence coverage. Some insurance companies no longer provide occurrence coverage. Residency programs throughout the country may provide occurrence coverage or claims-made coverage for their residents, but they seldom offer both at the same time.

Residents should determine the type of coverage provided during their residency. More important, if covered by a claims-made policy, they should make certain that tail coverage is provided by the residency program on completion of the residency. If tail coverage is not provided, residents leaving the program will be uninsured for subsequent claims arising from their practice during residency. Residents will then need to investigate the cost of such coverage with the insurer and arrange for its purchase. Residents also may explore the option of prior acts or "nose" coverage with another insurance carrier. The failure to purchase either tail or nose coverage in a timely manner after residency could jeopardize a resident's future insurability.

The Amount of Insurance Coverage

The amount of coverage provided for residents also is important. Obstetrics and gynecology is a high-risk specialty in the legal sense, and large jury awards are not uncommon. Residents should determine the amount of coverage provided by the program. Some programs may provide a specific amount of coverage, with a stated amount per incident and amount per year. If a program has $1 million/$3 million coverage, this means that residents are insured for up to $1 million per incident and up to $3 million per year.

Residents should not be too concerned if their program cannot specify an exact amount of incident and aggregate coverage for individual residents. The program may have a large combined aggregate coverage, which could provide insurance up to, for example, $25 million in a given year without a dollar limit per incident. In such a situation, residents should know the combined aggregate for the program.

It is impossible to state what is an adequate amount of insurance for residents in obstetrics and gynecology. Some states limit residents' liability by statute or by treating residents as state employees. Other states have patient compensation funds that decrease the amount of primary insurance that a residency program needs to buy. Residents have little power to negotiate with a residency program for a higher coverage amount, but they can and should know what is provided and how it relates to special circumstances in their state.

Restrictions on Liability Insurance Policies for Residents

Most residency liability policies have certain restrictions or exclusions. Residents should learn about these restrictions or exclusions, because liability coverage will not be provided for claims against residents caused by an activity that violates these restrictions or exclusions.

The most common exclusion is for "moonlighting" activities. It is not uncommon for residents to supplement their income by practicing in a department of obstetrics and gynecology or emergency room at another hospital or institution. In almost all cases, however, the residency liability insurance policy will not provide coverage for these activities. Residents who choose to moonlight should investigate whether the hospital or institution where they moonlight provides insurance coverage for residents. If not, residents should purchase professional liability insurance coverage for these activities or be willing to run the risk of being uninsured for claims resulting from moonlighting practice. Again, residents should investigate the type of coverage available. If it is claims-made coverage, residents should look closely at the cost of purchasing tail coverage before deciding to moonlight.

Future Considerations for Residents

Even if residents are provided with coverage that insures them for an adequate amount for all claims during residency, there is another insurance issue of some concern. It is called "surcharging or experience rating." Because of consumer demands and the impression that the medical professional liability crisis has been caused by a small number of bad physicians, some insurance companies and state insurance commissioners have adopted surcharging or experience-rating plans for medical professional liability insurance. Although these plans vary, all assess points against a physician for the number of medical professional liability claims experienced, the outcome of the claims, and the amounts paid on behalf of the physician. When a physician exceeds a certain point threshold, that physician is typically assessed an additional premium greater than the nominal premium for the specialty.

Unfortunately, it is not uncommon for a plaintiff's attorney to file claims against all health care practitioners whose names appear in a plaintiff's medical record, including all residents. Residents who have experienced a number of medical professional liability claims during residency should investigate the surcharging or experience-rating practices of prospective insurance carriers or states before going into private practice. Residents who neglect to make these inquiries may find that insurance is unavailable or prohibitively expensive.

Residents should not rely solely on the residency employment contract for evidence of medical professional liability insurance. An informal survey of residency employment contracts by ACOG's Department of Professional Liability/Risk Management revealed that many of these contracts contained nothing about professional liability insurance coverage. Those that addressed the issue in the contracts often did so in vague or confusing ways. Many contracts contained nothing about the type of coverage provided, whether tail coverage was provided for residents, the amount of coverage, or restrictions and exclusions to the coverage.

Residents always should attempt to obtain a copy of the master liability insurance policy for the residency program or a written statement or certificate of the coverage provided to residents. Claims can be made years after residency is completed. Some residency programs and some insurance companies may purge their files, and residents may be required at some point to prove that they have coverage for a claim. Residents should make a point of obtaining evidence of insurance for each year of residency, and they should save this evidence in their personal files indefinitely.

Professional Liability Insurance Coverage After Residency

Purchasing professional liability insurance is one of the most important and most expensive decisions physicians will ever make. A thoughtful consideration and examination should be made before purchasing professional liability insurance. It is essential to know the exact type of policy being purchased. Physicians should check with their state insurance department for information about the carrier, including the reputation, history, and financial stability of traditional registered insurance carriers. Physicians should know whether the insurance company is a licensed and admitted carrier in the state in which they are going to practice, and whether it participates in the state guaranty fund. Guaranty funds have been established by law in every state to protect policyholders in case an insurer becomes insolvent or is unable to meet its financial obligations. Physicians should be aware that guaranty funds cover only admitted carriers, not other vehicles for insuring against medical liability claims, such as trust or risk retention groups or risk purchasing groups. A state's insurance insolvency fund will not provide protection for unregistered insurance companies. A risk retention group is required only to register with the insurance department in its state of incorporation. Self-insurance funds may not have to register at all.

As a part of this investigation, physicians should attempt to obtain a sample copy of the policy and should thoroughly know and understand its contents. It is a good idea for physicians to have a personal attorney review the sample policy. Physicians also should ask about the company's underwriting criteria for termination, cancellation, nonrenewal, and surcharges, and consider how those criteria would affect practice. A cheaper premium is not always the better buy. In addition, when considering purchasing insurance from a nontraditional insurance mechanism, physicians should check with their hospitals to see if the insurance being offered satisfies its requirements for members of the medical staff.

Types of Liability Insurance Coverage

The two basic types of professional liability insurance, occurrence coverage and claims-made coverage, were discussed previously. The descriptions of these types of insurance and the caveats about them outlined for the residency period also apply to insurance purchased after residency. In addition, there is a variation on claims-made coverage with which physicians should be familiar: claims-paid coverage.

The key differences between claims-made coverage and claims-paid coverage are the timing of when the coverage begins and the definition of what the insurance carrier considers a "claim." In claims-made coverage, a claim is defined as a formal demand for money or the filing of a lawsuit. Yet many claims-made policies require insureds to report all incidents. It is important to review the policy carefully to see how the term claim is defined and to check notice requirements for reporting claims.

Under a claims-paid policy, everything surrounding a claim, including the incident of alleged medical professional liability, the filing of a lawsuit, the reporting of the lawsuit to the carrier, and the payment of the claim must all occur within the same policy year. Premiums for claims-paid coverage are based on what the carrier expects to pay out for the year the policy is in effect. Premiums for claims-paid insurance typically are cheaper than claims-made coverage. However, if the carrier did not adequately predict the pay-out in claims for any given year, the carrier typically has reserved the right to assess its insureds to pay off the carrier's losses. Tail coverage also needs to be purchased if a resident leaves the carrier, and the cost of such coverage is frequently 2 to 10 times the amount of the last premium, and usually is based on the number of years in practice and claims experience.

Exclusions from Liability Insurance Coverage

Every medical liability insurance policy has an *exclusions* section, which outlines specific circumstances under which coverage will not apply. Some of these exclusions are liability assumed by contractual agreements with health maintenance organizations (HMOs), actions by employees of the medical practice other than the physician, or practicing outside of certain standards of care mandated by the insurer. Some liability policies exclude coverage of defense costs, or limit such costs. Most policies exclude coverage for claims arising from sexual misconduct, practicing under the influence of alcohol or illegal drugs, antitrust violations, criminal or grossly negligent acts, and libel or slander. Coverage usually is excluded for lawsuits that arise from incidents that do not involve rendering patient care. There are other areas that might be excluded from coverage, such as punitive damages in some states, so physicians should read and understand these areas of exclusion.

Options for Settlement of Claims

Another part of the professional liability insurance policy about which physicians need to be knowledgeable is how much control the insurance carrier has over whether, how, and when to settle a claim with or without the physician's consent. Without a clause guaranteeing the physician's *right-to-consent-to-settlement* an insurance company can settle a claim regardless of the insured's wishes. Instead of a *right-to-consent-to-settlement* clause, a policy may contain a *hammer clause*. This clause spells out the monetary consequences for the insured physician in the event that a physician refuses an insurer's settlement recommendation and an ensuing trial results in a higher award. These issues may be addressed by *options* written into the policy. Physicians should carefully read these *options* and try to negotiate the inclusion or exclusion of these options, as appropriate.

Types of Insurance Carriers

Professional liability insurance is available through a variety of sources all of which are designed to distribute, or spread, the risk among those whom they insure. Professional liability insurance carriers can be commercial companies, association-owned (or captive) companies, mutuals, risk retention groups, or nonprofit trusts. They may be owned by physician groups, sponsored by state medical societies, or self-insuring organizations. Insurers also vary in terms of how they are organized who owns or controls them, their financial stability, and whether or how they are regulated by state laws.

In addition to these traditional types of insurance carriers, a number of different insurance mechanisms have come into existence in recent years. Two such nontraditional mechanisms are risk retention groups and purchasing groups.

A risk retention group is a special insurance entity which is limited to individuals or organizations engaged in similar activities with similar or related liability exposure. Risk retention groups can be readily identified because they are required by law to use the phrase "risk retention group" in their name. Members are required to share a common business, trade, or profession. For example, physicians could form a risk retention group for professional liability insurance, but, by definition, physicians and engineers would not be permitted to form such a group.

Risk retention groups pose several caveats for consumers. Unlike traditional insurance, they are required to comply with state insurance laws only in the state in which the group is formed or licensed. Because the activities of a risk retention group are primarily regulated by the state in which it is licensed, risk retention groups often are incorporated in states with loose insurance regulations.

Once a risk retention group is licensed, it can then offer insurance in other states. This means that the nonlicensing state's insurance department would have only limited jurisdiction, and a risk retention group would not be subject to all of the state's insurance or securities laws. When a traditional insurance company becomes insolvent, a state's guaranty fund provides at least some of the original coverage to the insureds. Risk retention groups, however, only participate in a guaranty fund in the state in which they are licensed.

Purchasing groups do not write insurance; they only purchase insurance from traditional or nontraditional carriers, including risk retention groups. It is easy to establish a purchasing group because they are exempt from many existing state requirements regarding group insurance laws. They also are exempt from insurance financial regulations by states.

The Liability Insurance Carrier–Physician Relationship

Like any relationship or contract, each party to the insurance policy has responsibilities and obligations to the other. The insurance company agrees to accept financial responsibility on behalf of the insured for payment of any judgment or settlement up to a specific monetary limit in return for a fee (premium). In addition, the company is financially responsible for investigating a claim, negotiating a settlement, and defending the insured.

Physicians must know what is stated in their professional liability policies and what requirements and obligations are placed on them. Physicians may be required to notify their carriers as soon as a claim is made or suspected. Many physicians are afraid that their premiums will increase or their policies will be canceled because of early notification of an incident or claim. This may be a legitimate concern; however, there are advantages to early notification. Early notification aids in early evaluation and preparation of a case, which in turn improves the chances of a successful defense should an actual claim develop. Such action affords the insurance company and the defense counsel the opportunity to begin collecting and recording facts early and evaluating the case for merit. In some instances, the defense attorney may be able to negotiate an early settlement with the patient before litigation begins. It is important to remember that any written or recorded information given to the insurance company is subject to discovery by the plaintiff. Therefore, physicians should direct all communication to the defense attorney once one has been assigned to the case, because information given to defense attorneys is not discoverable.

Physicians have a duty to cooperate with their insurance companies in the defense of their cases, and failure to do so may cause the policy to be voided. Therefore, to meet the obligation to cooperate with their assigned defense attorneys, physicians must candidly and in good faith discuss all aspects of the case so that there are no surprises. An insurance company may, by the terms of the policy, have the right to settle a claim without the physician's consent. However, most carriers exercise this right sparingly and usually ask for consent to any settlement. Physicians may be faced with other pressures to settle, including the potential expense, the time lost from their practices, and the mental and emotional strain associated with litigation. Physicians may realize that there is more at risk than initially anticipated and want to settle. All of these pressures should be discussed thoroughly with the insurance carrier and defense attorney before arriving at a decision to make a settlement offer. If the defense counsel recommends settling, physicians should ask for an explanation justifying a settlement. They also should ask to be given the opportunity to concur in any settlement offers, even if the carrier has a right to settle without their consent. A good rapport between the physician, the carrier, and the defense attorney will aid in achieving such requests.

Another major concern of physicians is the possible need for personal defense counsel. The typical professional liability policy gives the insurer the right to select counsel and control the defense of a claim. However, there may be instances when personal defense counsel is warranted. If insurers feel that physicians' coverage is not adequate, they will be advised of the right to obtain personal defense counsel at their own expense to protect personal financial exposure. Physicians in this situation would be well advised to do so.

Another problem can arise regarding whether physicians are covered for an incident. This would typically arise as a question about whether a physician was insured for a particular procedure or whether the policy was in effect at the time of the incident. In such circumstances, the carrier will send a "reservation-of-rights" letter in which it will agree to defend the physician but reserve the right to contest the coverage problem after the medical professional liability case is resolved. With the increasing popularity of "gyn-only" policies, this issue may become one of increasing importance to the specialty of obstetrics and gynecology. These policies specifically state what constitutes "gyn-only" practice. Engaging in procedures that go beyond the scope of that definition may create problems. Physicians who receive a reservation-of-rights letter are strongly advised to retain their own personal defense counsels.

It is vital to keep the actual insurance policy after it has expired. Insurance companies may purge their records after a number of years without regard to the statute of limitations. Physicians may be required to prove to the company that they were insured for an incident, and the policy itself is the best evidence. (See the glossary for definitions of professional liability insurance terms.)

CHAPTER 12

Examples of Government Requirements Affecting Medical Practice

Patient Screening and Transfer (Emergency Medical Transfer in Active Labor Act)
　Interhospital Care and Transfer
　Referring Hospital
　Receiving Hospital
　Transport Team
　Air Transport
　Education

Privacy and Accountability of Individually Identifiable Health Information
　Transactions
　Security
　Privacy
　　Patient Consent
　　Privacy Officer
　　Minimum disclosure
　　Patient Inspection of Information

Fraud and Abuse

Medical Office Environment
　Occupational Safety and Health Administration Regulations
　Americans with Disabilities Act
　Clinical Laboratory Improvement Amendments of 1988

As a provider of health care, physicians should be aware that there are many federal and state guidelines and regulations that affect the practice of medicine. Some of the federal government regulations that commonly affect the provision of health care services are discussed in this chapter. For more complete information, physicians should contact their state medical societies, the appropriate state or federal regulatory agency, or their attorneys.

Patient Screening and Transfer (Emergency Medical Transfer in Active Labor Act)

Specific federal legal requirements apply to patient screening in emergency rooms and the transfer of patients, including those in labor (Emergency Medical Transfer in Active Labor Act), by Medicare-participating hospitals. It is essential that institutions and health care practitioners understand their obligations under the law. Even hospitals that are not capable of handling high-risk deliveries or high-risk infants and have written transfer agreements must meet all the screening, treatment, and transfer requirements before transferring a patient.

Interhospital Care and Transfer

Federal law mandates that all Medicare-participating hospitals provide an appropriate medical screening examination for any individual who seeks medical treatment at an emergency department and places strict requirements on the transfer of these patients. Both the facilities and the professionals providing care must understand their obligations under the laws regarding patient transfer.

Interhospital transport is appropriate and recommended if services and staff are not available at the referring facility to care for the patient. Prior to transport, the hospital must still meet the screening, treatment, and transfer requirements. Many legal details of transport are not well defined, but all involved parties are charged with a number of responsibilities. Some of these include:

- Each transport system must comply with the standards and regulations established by local, state, and federal agencies.
- Informed consent for transfer, transport, and admission at the receiving hospital should be obtained before the transport team moves the patient.
- Formal agreements between hospitals should be developed to outline procedures and responsibilities for patient care.
- Relevant patient identification should be provided for the patient to wear during transport.
- Patient care guidelines, orders, and verbal communication are to be used to care for the patient during transport.

Referring Hospital

The referring hospital and physician are responsible for the care of patients until they arrive at the receiving hospital. The referring physician is responsible for evaluating and stabilizing the patient before transfer. Both the referring physician and the hospital should understand the transport system, including how to gain access to and appropriately use its services. When transferred, each patient should be accompanied by a form that includes general information about the patient, reason for transfer, transport mode, and medical information that may enhance understanding of the patient's needs or problems.

Receiving Hospital

The receiving hospital is responsible for the overall coordination of the transport program. It should ensure that the interhospital transport system is organized to provide appropriate care for the transported patient. Contingency plans should be established to avoid a shortage of beds for patients requiring transport. The receiving center is responsible for providing consultant physicians with the following abilities:

- Communication capability 24 hours per day
- Reports that describe the patient's condition and planned therapy

- Summary of the hospital course and recommendations for ongoing care after discharge

Transport Team

The transport team should have the necessary expertise to provide supportive care for a wide variety of emergency conditions that can arise during transport. The composition of the team should be consistent with the expected level of medical needs of the patient being transported. The transport unit should:

- Provide rapidly available vehicles and staff
- Provide communication between the transport team and the receiving hospital
- Coordinate all levels of transfer (air and ground)
- Maintain sufficient patient care equipment for safe transport, the most necessary of which will include:
  - Physiologic function monitors (eg, heart rate, blood pressure, temperature, respiratory rate, transcutaneous oxygen assessments)
  - Resuscitation and support equipment (eg, intravenous pumps, suction apparatus, ventilators)
  - Medical gas tanks
  - Functional capabilities to support electrical equipment

Air Transport

Hospital-based equipment may develop flaws in flight and affect the safety of the patient. All equipment should be tested regularly to ensure accuracy and safety during air transport. The following agencies can offer assistance in choosing or testing the medical equipment used during air transport:

- The U.S. Army Aeromedical Research Laboratory, Fort Rucker, Alabama
- Armstrong Laboratory, Brooks Air Force Base, Texas
- Association of Air Medical Services, Pasadena, California
- Emergency Care Research Institute, Plymouth Meeting, Pennsylvania
- Federal Aviation Administration, Washington, DC

Education

An education program that informs users and the public about the capabilities of the interhospital transfer service is fundamental to the success of the operation. Outreach education should reinforce cooperation between all referring hospitals, and the providers in the system should know about the clinical capabilities and special resources of each institution. A mechanism should exist to rapidly inform all participants in the transport program about new changes or procedures.

Privacy and Accountability of Individually Identifiable Health Information

The Health Insurance Portability and Accountability Act of 1996 (HIPAA) was passed to ensure that people have access to health insurance when they leave a job or if they have preexisting medical conditions, and to control the flow of sensitive patient information in the electronic age. There are a number of health care provisions contained in HIPAA and it is vital that physicians are familiar with them. There are several parts of HIPAA that will affect how a medical practice operates.

Transactions

On August 17, 2000, federal regulations went into effect that standardize and simplify how health information is electronically stored and transmitted. Everyone involved in storing or transmitting claims data electronically must use the same formats and code sets by October 2002. Contracts should require vendors to comply with all HIPAA transactions, security, and privacy regulations.

Security

Final security regulations had not been released as of December 2001, but it is expected that they will be very similar to the preliminary regulations released in August 1998. These regulations will outline what must be done to prevent unauthorized disclosure of protected health care information. The security measures will include the use of electronic signatures, as well as safeguards for physical storage, transmission, and access to the health information of individuals. Requirements will be "scalable," meaning that precautions should be appropriate for the size of the organization. A summary of the preliminary security regulation is available on the Internet at http://aspe.os.dhhs.gov/admnsimp/bannerps.htm#security.

Privacy

Final privacy regulations went into effect April 14, 2001. Physician group practices have until April 14, 2003, to comply with the regulations.

The regulations apply to health plans, health care clearinghouses, and health care providers including hospitals and physicians—referred to as covered entities in the regulations. The privacy regulations cover protected health information, which includes all individually identifiable health information in any form—paper, electronic, and oral and include the following key components:

Patient Consent

Physicians must obtain written consent from the patient to use or disclose the protected health information for payment or treatment. Exceptions include emergencies and situations where the provider is legally obligated to provide care to the patient.

Privacy Officer

Covered entities, including physician medical practices, must designate a privacy official to develop and implement privacy policies and procedures. Small offices may assign this duty to an existing staff person. All staff must be trained on the regulations and the associated policies and procedures.

Minimum Disclosure

Covered entities must only disclose the minimum amount necessary to achieve the purpose of the disclosure, with the exceptions of disclosures to the patient or for treatment. Policies and procedures must be implemented to limit the information disclosed. Physicians are not limited in their disclosures to other providers for treatment purposes.

Patient Inspection of Information

Patients have the right to inspect and receive a copy of their protected health information. Physicians may charge a reasonable cost-based fee for copying the information.

There are stiff penalties for violating these regulations. A covered entity can be fined up to $100 per incident for accidental disclosure of personal health information, up to $25,000 per year, and purposeful misuses could result in fines of up to $250,000 and 10 years in prison. A summary of the rights and protections available under the privacy rule and more detailed information is available on the Internet at www.hhs.gov.

Fraud and Abuse

In medical practice, the phrase "fraud and abuse" generally refers to knowingly making efforts to obtain payment for services that were not provided as presented or that were not medically necessary. All physicians have the responsibility to:

- Accurately document the services provided. Documentation must be complete and legible.
- Ensure that bills are accurately coded and accurately reflect the services provided, as documented in the medical records.
- Ensure that the services or items provided are reasonable and necessary. There must be no incentives for unnecessary services.

There are several federal criminal and civil statutes related to fraud and abuse in health care. Physicians should consult legal experts to learn how the various laws specifically impact their practices.

Among the federal government's primary weapons for fighting fraud are the False Claims Acts (FCA), a criminal statute, and its civil counterpart. Both of these Acts have been used to prosecute Medicare and Medicaid fraud. It is a violation of these statutes to present a claim to a federal health care program that is knowingly false or fraudulent. A conviction under the criminal FCA carries both a fine and imprisonment of up to 5 years. Under the civil FCA, the government can assess treble damages and $5,000–10,000 in penalties for each false or fraudulent claim filed.

The Antikickback Statute prohibits a physician from knowingly and willfully receiving or paying kickbacks, bribes, or other remuneration for a referral or to influence the purchase or the sale of health care related goods or services. If found guilty, a physician will be convicted of a felony and fined up to $25,000 or imprisoned for up to 5 years or both.

The physician self-referral prohibitions (Stark I and Stark II) do not allow physicians to refer patients to entities for designated health services if they or their immediate family members have an ownership, investment, or compensation relationship with the entity. The law only pertains to services paid for by federal health care programs. There are numerous exceptions to the prohibitions. Physicians who violate the statute may be fined up to $15,000 per improper claim and face exclusion from Medicare and Medicaid. Physicians who enter into an arrangement with another entity that they know or should know circumvents the referral restrictions may be subject to a civil penalty of up to $100,000 per arrangement, as well as be excluded from Medicare and Medicaid. Even if false claims are submitted inadvertently or unknowingly, overpayments discovered during an audit must be repaid—and these repayments can hit a practice very hard if they have occurred for several years.

All medical practices and facilities should evaluate and monitor their adherence to Medicare and Medicaid billing requirements. The Department of Health and Human Service's Office of the Inspector General recommends that physician practices and medical facilities implement plans to ensure compliance with federal health care program requirements. This compliance guidance is available on the Office of the Inspector General's web site www.oig.hhs.gov.

Medical Office Environment

There are many federal laws and regulations impacting the physician's office environment. Three that will be mentioned here are the Occupational Safety and Health Administration (OSHA) Regulations on Occupational Exposure to Bloodborne Pathogens, the Americans with Disabilities Act (ADA), and the Clinical Laboratory Improvement Amendments of 1988 (CLIA). Physicians should become aware of their responsibilities in these areas (see also ACOG's *Guidelines for Women's Health Care*, 2nd Edition).

Occupational Safety and Health Administration Regulations

The Occupational Safety and Health Administration has the responsibility for developing and implementing job safety and health standards and regulations which apply to all employers and employees. In 1991, OSHA issued regulations on occupational exposure to bloodborne pathogens that are designed to minimize the transmission of human immunodeficiency virus (HIV), hepatitis B virus (HBV), and other potentially infectious materials in the workplace. The regulations cover all employees in physician offices, hospitals, medical laboratories, and other health care facilities where workers could be "reasonably anticipated" as a result of performing their job duties to come into contact with blood and other potentially infectious materials. For more information, contact the U.S. Department of Labor, OSHA Office of Public Affairs, at (202) 693-1999 or visit www.dol.gov.

Americans with Disabilities Act

The ADA protects individuals with disabilities against discrimination in certain critical areas of daily living. These areas include protections for health services, employment, communication, public accommodations, education, and transportation. Disability is defined broadly to include both physical and mental impairments that substantially limit one or more major life activities of an individual. A person who has a record of either a physical or a mental impairment or a person who is regarded as having such an impairment also is considered as having a disability. Because a physician's office is considered a "public accommodation" under the ADA, physicians must understand their obligations to accommodate disabled patients as well as disabled employees. For information about ADA compliance, call the ADA Information Line at 800-514-0301 or visit www.usdoj.gov.

Clinical Laboratory Improvement Amendments of 1988

The Clinical Laboratory Improvement Amendments of 1988 requires federal oversight for all laboratories, including physician offices, that perform tests that examine human specimens for the diagnosis, prevention, or treatment of any disease, impairment of health, or health assessment. All physician offices that conduct any such tests should have registered their laboratory with the Centers for Medicare and Medicaid Services (CMS) (formerly the Health Care Financing Administration) and obtained an appropriate certificate. The Centers for Medicare and Medicaid Services maintains a registry of laboratories that it has determined to be not in conformance with CLIA regulations. This can be obtained from one of the CMS regional offices or through its national office. The majority of obstetrician–gynecologists' offices have either certificates of waiver or certificates for provider-performed microscopy procedures. For more information on CLIA requirements, contact the regional CMS CLIA offices or www.cms.gov.

CHAPTER 13

Physician Reporting Requirements and Profiling

The Data Banks
  National Practitioner Data Bank
  Healthcare Integrity and Protection Data Bank

State Physician Profiling

The Data Banks

The National Practitioner Data Bank (NPDB) and the Healthcare Integrity and Protection Data Bank (HIPDB) are tools used to collect and dispense information on various actions taken against health care practitioners. General descriptions of the Data Banks are included in this chapter. Additional information is available from the Data Banks Helpline at 800-767-6732 or www.npdb-hipdb.org and contained in both the *National Practitioner Data Bank Guidebook* and the *Healthcare Integrity and Protection Data Bank Guidebook*.

National Practitioner Data Bank

The National Practitioner Data Bank contains information on adverse licensure actions, clinical privileges actions, and professional society membership actions taken against physicians and dentists. It also collects reports of medical professional liability payments made on behalf of health care practitioners. Congress clearly did not consider a settlement payment as evidence of negligence. The law states: "A payment in settlement of a medical malpractice action or claim shall not be construed as creating a presumption that medical malpractice has occurred." Rather, it was felt that hospitals and licensing boards should be aware of medical professional liability payment information to use as they saw fit in their review processes. State licensing and disciplinary boards have access to NPDB information, as do hospitals and other health care entities that conduct peer review on members and prospective members of their medical staff, employees, and potential employees.

Hospitals are required to check the NPDB when considering applicants to their medical staff and every 2 years for members of their medical staff. Hospitals are not required to check the NPDB about medical residents, interns, or staff fellows, even though these individuals may hold licenses to practice medicine. They are considered trainees in supervised programs of graduate medical education. Hospitals are required, however, to check the NPDB when residents or interns are appointed to the medical staff or are granted clinical privileges beyond the aegis of the residency program, such as moonlighting in the emergency room.

The public does not have access to the NPDB. Attorneys have access when a hospital and a physician are being sued and the hospital did not check the NPDB about that physician as required. The information acquired from the NPDB in these circumstances can only be used in that particular lawsuit and only against the hospital. There also are strong penalties for breaches of confidentiality in the law.

The law requires the reporting of all payments, within 30 days of the payment, made on behalf of a physician or licensed health care practitioner to settle or satisfy a judgment in a medical professional liability case. This includes payments on behalf of residents. However, medical professional liability payments made by individuals on their own behalf are not reportable. Payment information that is reportable to the NPDB also must be reported to the state medical board in the state where the incident occurred. If there is no payment made on behalf of the physician, no report is required. The law's definition of a medical professional liability action is very broad. It includes written complaints or demands for compensation even if no formal action is ever filed. For example, if a refund of a fee results from a written demand for monetary payment for damages, the refund is reportable to the NPDB. Additionally, no report is filed if the physician is formally dismissed from the lawsuit before a settlement or judgment, unless the physician is dismissed from the lawsuit in consideration of a payment by a third party.

Whoever makes the payment on behalf of a physician or health care practitioner in satisfaction of a claim for medical negligence is required to notify the NPDB. This means that the hospital or insurance carrier will notify the NPDB of a payment made on behalf of a resident.

Most of the information that must be reported to the NPDB about a liability action is straightforward. It is submitted on the standard Medical Malpractice Payment Report form. Information on physicians includes their name, home and work addresses, date of birth, professional schools attended, and hospital affiliations. The report also includes the date of the alleged acts, the jurisdiction where the claim was filed, the date of judgment or settlement, the amount of payment, and the date of payment.

The report also contains a narrative of 2,000 characters or less, describing the acts or omissions that gave rise to the negligence claim and a classification of the claim according to codes established by the U.S. Department of Health and Human Services. This description is written by the entity (ie, hospital or insurance carrier) that makes a payment on the physician's behalf. Because of the subjective nature of this description, a prudent physician will discuss the description with the hospital or insurance carrier before the report is filed with the NPDB. If it becomes clear that the case is going to be settled, physicians should try to initiate a discussion about the description before settlement. It may be desirable to give the hospital or insurance company recommended language to use in the description. A physician's bargaining power will be strongest before the settlement. Once the payment is made, the deadline for reporting leaves little time for negotiating the language in the description. Physicians who think they are agreeing to settle a case for nuisance value because defending a case is too costly may be surprised to find that the NPDB report description says that they violated the standard of care.

The U.S. Department of Health and Human Services supports these discussions. If the practitioner is consulted about the report before the report is filed with the NPDB, it may decrease the likelihood of a dispute being filed about the report. The department also has acknowledged that some descriptions of cases settled for economic reasons may inaccurately reflect substandard care.

Physicians need to know what the report will say before agreeing to settle. Hospitals or insurance carriers should be encouraged to indicate that the case was without medical merit and was being settled for financial reasons, if this is true.

When the NPDB receives a report regarding a medical professional liability payment, it will send the physician a "Notification of a Report in the NPDB-HIPDB." Physicians should check the accuracy of all information at that time. They should not delay. A formal dispute with the NPDB must be filed within a certain period. There are specific procedures for disputing NPDB reports. When filing a dispute, a 2,000 character statement also may be entered into the NPDB describing the basis of the dispute and expressing the physician's view of the medical professional liability claim or the payment or both. Special care should be used in crafting the statement for the NPDB. This statement will be released, unedited, along with the NPDB report in response to queries. To dispute a NPDB report or file an appeal, physicians should contact the Helpline for detailed information on the procedures and physicians' rights and responsibilities. The toll free data banks' Helpline telephone number is 800-767-6732. The data banks' web site, www.npdb-hipdb.org, also is helpful.

The typical obstetrician–gynecologist has little to fear from the NPDB. Most credentialing bodies already require applicants to disclose more information than that contained in the NPDB reports. For example, most require applicants to disclose all open and closed medical professional liability claims, even if the claim was dropped or settled without payment, while the NPDB only contains reports on closed claims with payments attributable to a physician.

Healthcare Integrity and Protection Data Bank

The Healthcare Integrity and Protection Data Bank was created to help deter fraud and abuse in health insurance and health care delivery. Health care fraud burdens the United States with enormous financial costs and threatens health care quality and patient safety. Estimates of annual losses caused by health care fraud range from 3% to 10% of all health care expenditures—between $30 billion and $100 billion based on estimated 1997 expenditures of more that $1 trillion.

The HIPDB is a national health care fraud and abuse data collection program for the reporting and disclosure of certain final adverse actions taken against health care providers and suppliers. It is primarily a flagging system that may alert users that a comprehensive review of the practitioner, provider, or supplier's past actions may be prudent. The HIPDB is intended to augment, not replace, traditional forms of review and investigation, serving as an important supplement to a comprehensive and careful review of the practitioner, provider, or supplier's past actions. It is not currently accessible by the public.

As a nationwide flagging system, the HIPDB provides another resource to assist federal and state agencies (including law enforcement agencies), state licensing boards, and health plans in conducting extensive, independent investigations of the qualifications of the health care practitioners, providers, or suppliers, whom they seek to investigate, license, hire, or credential, or with whom they seek to contract or affiliate. Therefore, the information in the HIPDB should only alert federal or state agencies and health plans that there may be a problem with a particular practitioner, provider, or supplier. This information should always be considered together with other relevant data when evaluating the credentials of a healthcare practitioner, provider, or supplier.

The types of information filed with the HIPDB are licensure and certification actions, exclusions from participation in federal and state health care programs, criminal convictions related to health care, and civil judgments related to health care. Settlements in which no findings or admissions of liability have been made are not reported to this data bank. Also, medical professional liability claims are not reported to the HIPDB.

To be eligible to report to or query the HIPDB, an entity must be a health plan or a federal or state governmental agency. As with the NPDB, physicians can self-query the HIPDB. When the HIPDB processes a report, a "Report Verification Document" is sent to the reporting entity, and a "Notification of a Report in the Data Bank(s)" is sent to the subject. The report should be reviewed for accuracy. The subject of a report may add a 2,000 character statement to a report at any time. Both Data Banks have the same dispute process.

State Physician Profiling

Physicians should be aware that many states currently offer or are considering offering consumer access to "physician profiles." The stated purpose for collecting and releasing data is to allow consumers to make informed health care decisions.

Profiles differ in the types of information provided. In addition to practice information (primary work setting, address), sources may provide information on education, training, state medical board disciplinary actions, revocation or restriction of hospital privileges, disclosure of medical professional liability judgments, settled claims, and criminal convictions. Some states provide access via the Internet and a few by way of toll free telephone numbers.

Currently there is at least one organization collecting information on a national basis and selling it. For a fee, the Federation of State Medical Boards will send consumers a report on disciplinary actions taken against physicians. Collecting information for approximately 40 years, the Federation of State Medical Boards has just recently opened its files to the public.

REFERENCES

1. American College of Obstetricians and Gynecologists. Ethical issues related to expert testimony by obstetricians and gynecologists. In: Ethics in obstetrics and gynecology. Washington, DC: ACOG, 2002:38–39

2. American College of Obstetricians and Gynecologists. Ethical decision making in obstetrics and gynecology. In: Ethics in obstetrics and gynecology. Washington, DC: ACOG, 2002:1–6

3. American College of Obstetricians and Gynecologists. Informed refusal. ACOG Committee Opinion 237. Washington, DC: ACOG, 2000

4. American College of Obstetricians and Gynecologists. Ethical dimensions of informed consent. In: Ethics in obstetrics and gynecology. Washington, DC: ACOG, 2002:19–27

5. American College of Obstetricians and Gynecologists. Patient choice and the maternal–fetal relationship. In: Ethics in obstetrics and gynecology. Washington, DC: ACOG, 2002:61–63

6. American College of Obstetricians and Gynecologists. Sexual misconduct in the practice of obstetrics and gynecology: ethical considerations. In: Ethics in obstetrics and gynecology. Washington, DC: ACOG, 2002:89–91

7. American College of Obstetricians and Gynecologists. Code of professional ethics of the American College of Obstetricians and Gynecologists. Washington, DC: ACOG, 2002

8. American College of Obstetricians and Gynecologists. End-of-life decision making: understanding the goals of care. In: Ethics in obstetrics and gynecology. Washington, DC: ACOG, 2002:10–15

9. American College of Obstetricians and Gynecologists. Nonselective embryo reduction: ethical guidance for the obstetrician–gynecologist. In: Ethics in obstetrics and gynecology. Washington, DC: ACOG, 2002:53–56

10. American College of Obstetricians and Gynecologists. Sterilization of women, including those with mental disabilities. In: Ethics in obstetrics and gynecology. Washington, DC: ACOG, 2002:92–95

11. American College of Obstetricians and Gynecologists. Professional liability and its effects: report of a 1999 survey of ACOG's membership. Washington, DC: ACOG, 1999

12. American College of Obstetricians and Gynecologists. Professional liability and its effects: report of a 1987 survey of ACOG's membership. Washington, DC: ACOG, 1988

13. Freeman JM. Prenatal and perinatal factors associated with brain disorders. Bethesda, Maryland: National Institute of Child Health and Human Development, National Institute of Neurological and Communicative Disorders and Stroke, U.S. Department of Health and Human Services, Public Health Services, National Institutes of Health, April 1985. NIH Publication No. 85-1149

14. American College of Obstetricians and Gynecologists. Vaginal birth after previous cesarean delivery. ACOG Practice Bulletin 5. Washington, DC: ACOG, 1999

15. American College of Obstetricians and Gynecologists. Operative vaginal delivery. ACOG Practice Bulletin 17. Washington, DC: ACOG, 2000

16. American College of Obstetricians and Gynecologists. Shoulder dystocia. ACOG Practice Pattern 7. Washington, DC: ACOG, 1997

17. SEER cancer statistics review, 1973–1998 [serial online]. Available at http://www-seer.ims.nci.nih.gov/Publications/CSR1973_1998/. Retrieved October 22, 2001

18. Physician Insurers Association of America. Breast cancer study. Rockville, Maryland: PIAA, 1995

19. American College of Obstetricians and Gynecologists. Induction of labor. ACOG Practice Bulletin 10. Washington, DC: ACOG, 1999

Glossary

Medical–Legal Terms

Abandonment: Termination of a physician–patient relationship without reasonable notice and without an opportunity for the patient to acquire adequate medical care, which results in some type of damage to the patient.

Admissibility (in evidence): A characteristic of evidence that may properly be introduced in a legal proceeding. The determination as to admissibility is based on legal rules of evidence and is made by the trial judge or a screening panel.

Admissions: Statements by a party that are admissible in evidence as an exception to the hearsay rule. In a professional liability proceeding, an admission would typically be a statement of culpability by the defendant.

Affidavit: A voluntary, written statement of facts made under oath before an officer of the court or before a notary public. May be used at trial.

Affirmative Defense: An answer to a complaint that asserts a legal basis to excuse or foreclose liability (eg, expiration of statute of limitations, contributory negligence).

Allegation: A statement of a party to an action, made in a pleading, setting out what the party expects to prove.

Americans with Disabilities Act (ADA): Federal law which prohibits certain employers from discriminating against disabled persons when making decisions to hire, promote, or take other employment-related actions.

Answer: A legal document that contains a defendant's written response to a *Complaint* or *Declaration* in a legal proceeding. The *Answer* typically either denies the allegations of the plaintiff or makes new allegations as to why the plaintiff should not recover.

Appeal: The process by which a decision of a lower court is brought for review to a court of higher jurisdiction, typically known as an appellate court.

Appellate Court: The court that reviews trial court decisions. Appellate courts review the trial court proceedings and determine whether there were errors of law committed by the trial court. The appellate court does not make determinations respecting disputed questions of fact.

Bailiff: An officer of the court who is in charge of courtroom decorum, directs witnesses to the witness stand, and attends to the jurors.

Battery: The unauthorized and offensive touching of a person by another. In medical professional liability cases, battery is typically contact of some type with a patient who has not consented to the contact. Battery can be either a civil or a criminal offense.

Burden of Proof: The necessity or duty of affirmatively proving a fact or facts in a dispute. The plaintiff typically has the burden of proof.

Captain-of-the-Ship: A doctrine whereby the physician in charge of a medical team is liable for the negligent acts of all the members of the team.

Case: An action or cause of action; a matter in dispute; a lawsuit.

Case Law: Legal principles derived from judicial decisions. Case law differs from statutory law, which is enacted by legislatures.

Causation (or Cause): In negligence actions, a reasonable, proximate connection between a breach of duty and an injury sustained by the plaintiff.

Cause of Action: A set of alleged facts that a plaintiff uses to seek legal redress.

Clerk of the Court: The person who is responsible for the administrative functions of the court. During a trial, the clerk administers the oaths to the witnesses, receives and marks exhibits into evidence, and requests the verdict from the jurors.

Collateral Source Rule: A rule of law that prevents a court from subtracting any payments that the plaintiff has received from such sources as workmen's compensation, health insurance, government benefits, or sick pay benefits from the damage award.

Common Law: That body of case law that was passed down to the American colonies by the British court system and has been interpreted and refined by judicial decisions (or court decisions), as distinguished from statutory laws enacted by legislatures.

Comparative Negligence/Contributory Negligence: Affirmative defenses, one or the other of which is recognized in most jurisdictions.

- *Comparative negligence:* An affirmative defense that compares the negligence of the defendant with that of the plaintiff. The plaintiff may recover damages from a negligent defendant even if the plaintiff and defendant are equally at fault. It is only when the plaintiff's negligence is greater than the defendant's that there can be no recovery. The plaintiff's damages are decreased, however, by the percentage that his or her own fault contributed to the overall damage.

- *Contributory negligence:* An affirmative defense that prevents recovery against a defendant when the plaintiff's own negligence contributed to the injury, even though the defendant's negligence also may have contributed to the injury.

Complaint: A legal document that is the initial pleading on the part of the plaintiff in a civil lawsuit. A *Complaint* is sometimes known as a *Declaration*. The purpose of this document is to give a defendant notice of the alleged facts constituting the cause of action. The *Complaint* usually is attached to the *Summons*.

Compliance Program: A process designed to decrease or eliminate violations of federal requirements (eg, fraud and abuse, ADA, OSHA, EEOC).

Contingency Fee: A fee agreement between the plaintiff and the plaintiff's attorney, whereby the plaintiff agrees to pay the attorney a percentage of the damages recovered.

Counterclaim: A defendant's claim made in opposition to a claim made by the plaintiff (eg, malicious prosecution).

Court Reporter: A professionally trained stenographer who transcribes deposition or trial testimony.

Court Trial: A trial without a jury, wherein the judge determines the facts as well as the law.

Culpability: Being at fault, deserving reproach or punishment for some act or course of action. Culpability connotes wrongdoing or errors of ignorance, omission, or negligence.

Damages: The sum of money a court or jury awards as compensation for a tort. The law recognizes certain categories of damages. These categories often are imprecise and inconsistent. Variations exist among jurisdictions, and all are not strictly adhered to by the courts. The major categories are general, punitive, exemplary, and special damages.

- *General damages:* Typically intangible damages (eg, pain and suffering, disfigurement, interference with ordinary enjoyment of life).
- *Punitive or exemplary damages:* Damages awarded to the plaintiff to punish the defendant or act as a deterrent to others (eg, in cases of intentional tort or gross negligence).
- *Special damages:* Out-of-pocket damages (eg, medical expenses, lost wages, rehabilitation).

Declaration: See Complaint.

Deposition: A discovery procedure whereby each party may question in person the other party or anyone who may possibly be a witness. Depositions are conducted before the trial under oath and are admissible at trial under certain circumstances.

Directed Verdict: Ruling by the trial judge that, as a matter of law, the verdict must be in favor of a particular party. A verdict usually is directed because of a clear failure to meet the burden of proof, sometimes referred to as a failure to establish a prima facie case.

Discovery: Pretrial procedures to learn of evidence to minimize the element of surprise at the trial. These typically include *Interrogatories* and *Depositions* but also can include *Requests for Admission of Facts* and *Requests for Genuineness of Documents.*

Dismissal: A final disposition of an action, suit, motion, etc. To dismiss a motion is to deny it; to dismiss an appeal is to affirm the judgment of the trial court.

Due Care: The level of observation, awareness, and care owed by a physician to a patient.

Due Process: Legal procedures that have been established in systems or jurisprudence for the enforcement and protection of private rights. It often means simply a fair hearing or trial.

Duty: An obligation recognized by the law. A physician's duty to a patient is to provide the degree of care ordinarily exercised by physicians of the same or similar specialty practicing in the same community, or, increasingly, in the same country.

Evidence: Facts presented at trial through witnesses, records, documents, and concrete objects, for the purpose of proving or defending a case. Some examples of evidence are:

- *Circumstantial evidence:* Facts or circumstances that indirectly imply that the principal facts at issue actually occurred.
- *Demonstrative or real evidence:* The use of articles or objects rather than the statement of witnesses to prove a fact in question.
- *Direct evidence:* Evidence that is based on personal knowledge or observation and that, if true, proves a fact without inference or presumption.
- *Material evidence:* Evidence having some logical connection with the consequential facts.
- *Opinion evidence:* Testimony of an expert witness based on special training or background, rather than on personal knowledge of the facts in issue.
- *Prima facie evidence:* A level of proof that is sufficient to establish a fact, and if not rebuffed, becomes conclusive of the fact.

Expert Opinion: The testimony of a person who has special training, knowledge, skill, or experience in an area relevant to resolution of the legal dispute.

Federal Court: Federal courts are another system of trial and appellate courts like state courts. However, federal courts only accept certain types of cases. Medical professional liability cases generally are not filed in the federal courts unless a patient is from one state and the health care practitioner is from another state.

Fraud: An intentional misrepresentation of the truth or concealment of fact. Examples in medicine would be to exaggerate one's professional credentials to induce a patient to undergo tests or procedures or to misstate (upcode) diagnoses or treatment codes to maximize reimbursement.

Good Samaritan Statute: State laws enacted to encourage physicians, and others, to aid emergency victims. Statutes vary from state to state but generally grant immunity from liability for negligence when a caregiver acts gratuitously at the scene of an emergency and provides care in good faith. Because good samaritan laws are state-specific, physicians are urged to familiarize themselves with the law in effect in their jurisdiction.

Health Insurance Portability and Accountability Act of 1996 (HIPAA): Federal regulation affording some protection to individuals covered under group health insurance plans when that individual changes insurers. The object is to afford those insureds with preexisting conditions some protection against denial of coverage. Regulations concerning electronic claims transactions and privacy of patient information under HIPAA were finalized in 2001.

Hearsay: An out-of-court statement, made by another person, offered in court to prove the truth of the facts contained in the statement. Hearsay generally is not admissible. There are, however, exceptions to the hearsay rule, such as an admission against interest.

Hostile Witness: A witness whose position or viewpoint is adverse to that of the attorney who called him or her to the stand.

Hung Jury: A jury that cannot come to a decision that constitutes a verdict in its jurisdiction, frequently after lengthy deliberation. A hung jury results in a mistrial, which in most circumstances means the case will be retried before a new jury.

Hypothetical Question: A question that solicits the opinion of an expert witness at a trial or deposition based on a combination of assumptions and facts already introduced in evidence.

Impeachment: An attack on the credibility of a witness.

Informed Consent: A legal doctrine that requires a physician to obtain consent for treatment to be rendered or an operation to be performed; without an informed consent, the physician may be held liable for violation of the patient's rights, regardless of whether the treatment was appropriate and rendered with due care (*see* Battery).

Interrogatories: A discovery procedure in which one party submits a series of written questions to the opposing party, who must answer in writing under oath within a certain period. The answers are admissible at trial under certain circumstances.

Joint and Several Liability: A legal doctrine whereby each individual defendant is independently responsible for the entire amount of damages awarded against all defendants.

Judgment: The official decision in the record of a case, which is binding on the parties unless it is overturned or modified on appeal. A judgment typically consists of a finding in favor of one or more of the parties and an assessment of damages and costs.

Jury Trial: A trial in which 12 or fewer registered voters are impaneled to hear the evidence, determine the facts, and render a verdict. In most states, the verdict must be unanimous.

Litigation: The process of a court trial to determine legal issues.

Loss of Consortium: A claim for damages by the parent, child, or spouse of an injured party for the loss of care, comfort, society, and, when applicable, interference with sexual relations.

Maloccurrence: A bad medical outcome that is totally unrelated to the quality of care provided, ie, non-negligent.

Malpractice: Professional negligence. In medical terms, it is the failure to exercise that degree of care used by reasonably careful physicians in the same or similar circumstances of like qualifications. The failure to meet this acceptable standard of care must cause the patient injury.

Motion: Written or oral court plea requesting that a court or judge make an order or ruling affecting the lawsuit.

Negligence: Legal cause of action involving the failure to exercise due care expected of a reasonable person under the same or similar circumstances.

Party: A person or legal entity involved in a legal transaction or court proceeding (eg, a party to the contract or a party to the lawsuit).

Peer Review Organization (PRO): A government agency or an independent joint contract with a private group to review medical necessity, quality of care, or cost issues for Medicare and Medicaid patients, generally in connection with observation or inpatient hospital care or both.

Periodic Payments: Damages paid to a plaintiff over a period of time instead of in a lump sum all at once. If permitted by state law, periodic payments may be ordered when the damages exceed a certain amount.

Pleadings: Written documents filed in a lawsuit, through which the issues in dispute are identified and clarified, including the plaintiff's cause of action and the defendant's grounds of defense. Pleadings include the complaint, answer, and motions.

Preponderance of Evidence: The greater weight of evidence, or evidence that is more credible or convincing to the mind.

Prima Facie Case: A plaintiff's case with sufficient evidence to survive a motion for a directed verdict or a motion to dismiss by the defendant.

Privileged Communications: Confidential communication between individuals that attains a special legal status because of the nature of their relationship. Privileged communications include communications between attorney and client, husband and wife, physician and patient, and priest and penitent.

Proximate Cause: An act or omission that, unbroken by any intervening cause, produces an injury. In a medical professional liability case, failure to adhere to the standard of care must be the proximate cause of the injury to the patient.

Rebut: Refute; present opposing evidence or arguments.

Res Ipsa Loquitur: "The thing speaks for itself." A doctrine under which it can be demonstrated that the injury was caused by means under the defendant's exclusive control and would not have occurred in the absence of negligence. In medical professional liability cases, it allows a patient to prove his or her case without the necessity of an expert witness to testify that the defendant physician violated the standards of care. It is applicable only in those instances in which negligence is clear and obvious even to a layman, such as foreign object cases in which a surgeon leaves a sponge in the patient following surgery.

Reservation of Rights: An insurance term that refers to a carrier's conditional commitment to undertake the defense of a matter when there is a question as to the existence of coverage for an incident.

Respondeat Superior: "Let the master answer." The legal principle that makes an employer liable for civil wrongs committed by employees within the course and scope of their employment. In medical professional liability cases, this theory often is used to hold hospitals liable for the negligence of the staff employees and attending physicians responsible for residents.

Risk Management: Activities and strategies aimed at improving medical care while decreasing exposure to professional liability and financial loss.

Settlement: An agreement made between the parties to a lawsuit or a claim, which resolves their legal dispute.

Standard of Care: A term used in the legal definition of medical professional liability. A physician is required to adhere to the standards of practice of competent physicians, with comparable training and experience, in the same or similar circumstances.

Statute of Limitations: The period in which a plaintiff may file a lawsuit. Once this period expires, the plaintiff's lawsuit is barred if the defendant asserts the affirmative defense of the statute of limitations.

Stipulation: An agreement made by both parties to the litigation regulating any matter related to the case, proceeding, or trial. For instance, litigants can agree to extend the period for pleadings or to admit certain facts into evidence at trial.

Structured Settlement: Settlement agreement between the parties to a lawsuit or a claim in which the damages are paid to the plaintiff over a period of time, instead of in a lump sum all at once. These settlements usually are financed through the purchase of an annuity.

Subpoena: Court order requiring a witness to appear at a certain proceeding to give testimony or produce documents or both.

Summary Judgment: Granting of a judgment in favor of either party before trial. Summary judgment is granted only when there is no factual dispute and one of the parties is entitled to judgment as a matter of law.

Summons: A legal document that is attached to the *Complaint* or *Declaration* in a lawsuit. It orders the defendant or the defendant's attorney to file an *Answer* within a specified period.

Tort: A civil wrong, for which an action can be filed in court to recover damages for personal injury or property damage resulting from negligent acts or intentional misconduct. Four elements must be established to successfully litigate a tort claim: 1) a duty owed; 2) a breach of that duty; 3) an injury caused by the breach; and 4) damages.

Trier of Fact: The jury or, in the case of trial without jury, the judge.

Utilization Review or Utilization Management: A technique or program that evaluates the appropriateness, quality, and medical necessity of services provided to plan members. Can be administered by the hospital, health maintenance organizations, or insurance carriers. It can involve precertification of procedures and admissions, concurrent inpatient review, or retrospective review of patient medical records.

Verdict: The formal decision or finding made by a jury or judge. The verdict is in favor of the plaintiff or defendant, and damages usually are awarded when the verdict is in favor of the plaintiff.

Vicarious Liability: Civil liability for the actions of others. Physicians may be vicariously liable for the negligent acts of their employees committed within the scope of their employment (*see Respondeat Superior*). In the hospital setting, a surgeon may be vicariously liable for the negligent acts of all members of the surgical team (*see* Captain-of-the-Ship).

Work Product: Materials prepared by or for an attorney in anticipation of litigation. These materials are not subject to discovery.

Wrongful Birth: An action brought by parents who seek damages after the birth of an impaired child. The parents assert that they received inadequate medical care that led to the birth of a handicapped child and that if they had received proper genetic counseling or testing, the child's birth could have been avoided.

Wrongful Conception/Wrongful Pregnancy: An action brought by parents who seek damages for a healthy, but unplanned and unwanted child born as a result of failed sterilization, birth control, or abortion.

Wrongful Life: An action brought by an impaired child who contends that if his or her parents had been correctly counseled about likely birth defects, he or she would have never been conceived or would have been aborted.

Professional Liability Insurance Definitions and Terms

Captive Insurance Company: A company owned and controlled by those it insures, as when a hospital, hospital association, medical society, or medical specialty society establishes its own medical professional liability insurance company.

Claims-made Insurance Policy: A policy that covers only those claims that happen and are submitted during the term of the policy. Insurance coverage ceases on the date the policy is terminated unless extended reporting endorsement (tail) coverage is purchased. It is desirable that a claims-made policy includes a guarantee for purchase of an extended reporting endorsement and waiver of premium for the extended reporting endorsement in the event of death, disability, or retirement (an insurance company's definition of retirement may vary).

Commercial Insurance Company: A for-profit insurance company owned and controlled by stockholders (stock company) or policyholders (mutual company). Commercial or traditional insurance carriers are regulated by state law.

Extended Reporting Endorsement (Tail): A supplement or endorsement to a claims-made policy that provides coverage for any incident that occurred during the term of the claims-made policy but had not been brought as a claim by the time the insurer–policyholder relationship terminated. Tail coverage is purchased from a physician's existing carrier on termination or cancellation, and typically is provided on death, disability, or retirement.

Guaranty Fund: Established by law in every state, these funds usually are maintained by a state's insurance commission to protect policyholders in the event that a licensed insurer becomes insolvent or otherwise unable to meet its financial obligations. The funds usually are financed by assessments against all property and casualty insurers regulated by a state.

Joint Underwriting Association (JUA): A state-sponsored insurance company that has been created to make insurance available in tight market conditions. A JUA may or may not be required to provide professional liability insurance to all licensed physicians in the state, depending on state law. The solvency of the JUA typically is supported by assessments on insurance carriers licensed to do business in the state.

Liability Limits: The maximum sum or sums that an insurance company is obligated to pay for a settlement or judgment against an insured party. In medical professional liability policies, these limits generally are written with a limit per claim and a limit of aggregate liability for each year of coverage.

Occurrence Insurance Policy: An insurance policy that obligates the insurer to pay for claims which took place during the period covered by the policy, regardless of when the claim is filed. This type of policy does not require that the policyholder purchase an extended reporting endorsement (tail) on termination.

Physician-owned Insurance Company: A company typically owned and controlled by physicians, but not required to be a nonprofit corporation. It may be a captive insurance company.

Prior-acts (Nose): A supplement or endorsement to a claims-made insurance policy that may be purchased from a new carrier when a physician changes carriers and previously had a claims-made insurance policy. A prior-acts policy covers incidents that happened before the beginning of the new insurance relationship but that have yet to be reported or a claim brought forward. Prior-acts can be an alternative to an extended reporting endorsement (tail).

Reinsurance: Insurance purchased by a primary insurance carrier to reimburse it for settlements and judgments in excess of a specified limit.

Reservation of Rights: An insurance term that refers to a situation arising when there is a question as to whether there is coverage for an incident of medical professional liability.

Risk Purchasing Group (RPG): A group of people or entities with similar liability risks that are permitted under federal law to organize across state lines to buy insurance. The carrier that sells insurance to the group must be licensed in at least one state but need not be licensed in every state where a member of the group resides. The purchasing group itself does not have to be licensed in any state and thus are not subject to financial examination by state insurance departments nor are they covered by a state's guaranty fund.

Risk Retention Group (RRG): A special insurance entity that is limited to individuals or organizations engaged in similar activities with similar or related liability exposures; members must share a common business, trade, or profession. A RRG only is required to comply with state insurance laws in its state of incorporation. Once a group is licensed in one state, it can then sell insurance nationwide without fulfilling each state's licensure requirements. A RRG is allowed to contribute to a state's guaranty fund.

Self-insured or Self-funded Plan: A trust fund established to pay defense costs and liability losses on behalf of participants, typically established by a hospital, hospital association, or hospital corporation.

Underwriting: The selection process by which an insurance company evaluates the risk of loss and determines which of the risks (applicants) should be accepted. On an individual basis, underwriting also would determine the amounts and limits of coverage for individual applicants.

INDEX

A

Abbreviations, in medical records, 73
Abortion, moral opposition to, 57–58
Accountability, of individually identifiable health information, 95–97
Accuracy, of medical records, 73
ACOG. *See* American College of Obstetricians and Gynecologists
Act of commission, 5
Act of omission, 5
ADA. *See* Americans with Disabilities Act
Air transport, 94
Ambulatory care setting, risk management in, 47–49
American College of Obstetricians and Gynecologists (ACOG)
   1999 professional liability survey of, 60
   Code of Professional Ethics of, 56
   Committee on Ethics of, 41, 48
   Committee on Professional Liability of, 35–36
   Department of Professional Liability/Risk Management of, 80, 84

Americans with Disabilities Act (ADA), 99
Answer (legal document), 9–10
Antikickback Statute, 97
Assigned attorney, 8
Attending staff
   communication with residents, 46–47, 53
   vicarious liability and, 53–55

B

Body language, during testimony, 21
Borrowed servant doctrine, 53, 55–56
Bowie v. Hearn, 5
Breach of duty, 5
Breast cancer, missed diagnosis of, 63–64

C

Cancer, missed diagnosis of, 63–64
Captain-of-the-ship doctrine, 53
Causation, 5
Centan v. Cobb, 4
Centers for Medicare and Medicaid Services (CMS), 99–100
Cesarean delivery, 62

Chaperones, in examination rooms, 48
Chemically impaired physician, 58
Claim
   notice of, 9–11
   responding to, 10–11
   settlement of, 31–32
Claims-made coverage, 81–82, 85–86
Claims-paid coverage, 86
Clinical Laboratory Improvement Amendments of 1988, 99–100
Closing argument, 24
CMS. *See* Centers for Medicare and Medicaid Services
Code of Professional Ethics, of ACOG, 56
Committee on Ethics, of ACOG, 41, 48
Committee on Professional Liability, of ACOG, 35–36
Communication
   among health care team, 72
   between attending staff and residents, 46–47, 53
   with patient, 67–70
Complaint (legal document), 9–10
Compliance, notation in medical record, 74
Contributory negligence, 35
Corrections, to medical records, 76–77
Counteroffers, in settlements, 31
Cross-examination, 23

D

Damages, 6
Data banks, 102–106
Data Sharing System, 65
Declaration (legal document), 9–10
Defendant
   presence at depositions, 17
   and settlements, 29

Defendant's case, 23–24
Defense attorney
   and settlements, 29
   trust of, 20
Delivery methods, 61–63
Demands, in settlements, 31
Department of Professional Liability/Risk Management, of ACOG, 80, 84
Depositions, 13–17
   attendance at, 17
   conduct at, 16–17
   definition of, 13–14
   preparation for, 14–16
   procedure of, 14
Direct examination, 22–23
Directed verdict, 23
Disclosure
   degree of, 35–38
   minimum, 96
Discovery
   information subject to, 11, 89
   procedures for, 11–13
Documentation
   of informed consent, 34–35, 41–42
   medical records, 71–77
   of professional liability insurance, 90
   Request for Admission of Genuineness of Documents, 13
   at time of incident, 48
Drug dosages, in medical records, 73
Dual-servant doctrine, 55–56
Duty, 2–5

E

Early notification, to insurance carriers, 88–89
Electronic fetal monitoring, notation in medical record, 76

Emergency care, and informed consent, 39–40
Emergency Medical Transfer in Active Labor Act, 92
Emergency room
  attending staff–resident communication in, 47
  and refusal of patients, 3
  transfer of patients in, 3
Ethical considerations, of residents, 56–58
Evidence, and settlements, 30
Examination room, chaperones in, 48
Exemplary damages, 6
Experience-rating plans, 84
Expert witnesses
  and causation, 5
  and settlements, 30
  and standard of care establishment, 4–5

F

Failure to diagnose, 63–64
False Claims Acts (FCA), 97
Federation of State Medical Boards, 106
Follow-up care, 70
Forceps delivery, 63
Formal claim, settlement of, 31–32
Fraud and abuse, 97–98, 105–106

G

General damages, 6
Government requirements, 91–100
  on fraud and abuse, 97–98
  on individually identifiable health information, 95–97
  on medical office environment, 98–100
  on patient screening/transfer, 92–100

Guaranty funds, 85
Gyn-only insurance policies, 90

H

Hammer clause, in professional liability insurance, 87
Health care team, communication among, 72
Health Insurance Portability and Accountability Act of 1996 (HIPAA), 95
Healthcare Integrity and Protection Data Bank Guidebook, 102
Healthcare Integrity and Protection Data Bank (HIPDB), 102, 105–106
HIPAA. *See* Health Insurance Portability and Accountability Act of 1996
HIPDB. *See* Healthcare Integrity and Protection Data Bank
Hospital setting, attending staff–resident communication in, 46–47
Hospitals
  and interhospital patient transfer, 92–95
  risk management in, 44–47
  and settlements, 29
Hostile witness rule, 23
Hypothetical questions, 15

I

Inappropriate conduct, false charges of, 48
Incident management, 8–9, 31, 48
Incompetent physician, 58
Individually identifiable health information
  minimum disclosure of, 96
  patient access to, 96

Individually identifiable health information *(continued)*
  privacy and accountability of, 95–97
  security of, 95–96
  transactions involving, 95
Induction of labor, 65
Informed consent, 33–42
  communication and, 70
  degree of disclosure in, 35–38
  documentation of, 41–42
  process of, 38–40
  special circumstances in, 39–40
  state laws on, 38
Informed refusal, 40–41, 74
Instructions to the jury, 24
Insurance. *See* Professional liability insurance
Interhospital care/transfer, 92–95
Interrogatories, 12

J
Joint defense, 8
Judge, and settlements, 29
Jury, instructions to, 24

K
Keotnaka v. Zakaib, 35

L
Labor, induction of, 65
Laboratory tests/reports, notation in medical record, 76
Laparoscopy, 65
Largey v. Rothman, 38
Leading questions, 15
Legal proof, 2
Legibility, of medical records, 73–75
Liability. *See* Professional liability

M
Mediation, 28–29
Medicaid fraud, 97–98

Medical office environment, 98–100
Medical practice, government requirements affecting, 91–100
Medical probability, 5
Medical procedures, moral opposition to, 57–58
Medical professional liability lawsuit
  high-risk areas for obstetricians and gynecologists, 59–65
  pretrial stage of, 7–17
  settlement stage of, 27–32
  trial stage of, 19–25
Medical records, 71–77
  accuracy of, 73
  comprehensiveness of, 73–74
  corrections to, 76–77
  informed consent notes in, 42
  legibility of, 73–75
  objectivity of, 75
  and risk management, 45
  tampering with, 11, 76
  timeliness of, 75–76
Medicare
  and fraud, 97–98
  and patient screening/transfer, 92
Melendez v. Hospital for Joint Diseases, 32
Minimum disclosure, 96
Minors, and informed consent, 39–40
Moonlighting, insurance restrictions on, 83
Moral opposition, to medical procedures, 57–58
Mozingo v. Pitt County Memorial Hospital, 55

N
National Institutes of Health (NIH), 61
National Practitioner Data Bank Guidebook, 102

National Practitioner Data Bank
(NPDB), 31, 102–105
National standard of care, and risk
management, 45
Negligence, 2
Neonatal death, 61
Neurologically impaired infant, 61
NIH. *See* National Institutes of
Health
Notice of a claim, 9–11
Notification of a Report in the
National Practitioner Data
Bank–Healthcare Integrity
and Protection Data Bank,
104, 106
NPDB. *See* National Practitioner
Data Bank
Nursing notes, notation in medical
record, 74

O

Objectivity, of medical records, 75
Obstetrics and gynecology, high-
risk areas for litigation in,
59–65
Occupational Safety and Health
Administration (OSHA),
98–99
Occurrence coverage, 81–82, 85–86
On-call duty, 49
Opening statements, 22
Operative vaginal delivery, 62–63
Options, in professional liability
insurance, 87
OSHA. *See* Occupational Safety and
Health Administration
Outpatient setting
attending staff–resident communi-
cation in, 47
risk management in, 47–49
Outreach education, on interhospital
patient transfer, 95

P

Patient
capacity to understand, 34
communication with, 67–70
consent, in privacy of health information, 96
inspection of information, 96
screening, 92–95
transfer, interhospital, 92–95
air transport, 94
outreach education for, 95
receiving hospital in, 93–94
referring hospital in, 93
transport team in, 94
Patient viewpoint standard, in
informed consent, 36–38
Perjury, 76
Personal attorney, 8, 89
Physician
communication with residents,
46–47, 53
incompetent, 58
profiling, 106
reporting requirements, 102–106
self-referral prohibitions, 97–98
vicarious liability and, 53–55
Physician Insurers Association of
America (PIAA)
breast cancer claims to, 64
laparoscopic claims to, 65
Physician–patient relationship
communication in, 68–70
and duty, 2–3
refusal to establish, 3, 56
PIAA. *See* Physician Insurers
Association of America
Plaintiff, presence at depositions, 16
Plaintiff's attorney, and settlements,
29
Plaintiff's case, 23
Plaintiff's rebuttal, 24
Postverdict activity, 25

Prenatal and Perinatal Factors Associated with Brain Disorders, 61
Preponderance of the evidence, 2
Pretrial stage
   of medical professional liability lawsuit, 7–17
   witness preparation in, 20–21
Privacy, of individually identifiable health information, 95–97
Privacy officer, 96
Professional liability, elements of, 1–6
Professional Liability and Its Effects: Report of a 1999 Survey of ACOG's Membership, 60
Professional liability insurance, 79–90
   coverage after residency, 85–90
      carrier–physician relationship, 88–90
      carriers of, 87–88
      exclusions from, 86
      settlement options in, 87
      types of, 85–86
   coverage during residency, 10, 80–84
      amount of, 82–83
      future considerations for, 83–84
      restrictions on, 83
      types of, 81–82
   documentation of, 90
   and settlements, 29, 31
Professional liability lawsuit, definition of, 2
Professional negligence, 2
Profiling, of physicians, by state, 106
Punitive damages, 6

Q

Questions, in cross-examination, 15

R

Refusal of care. *See* Informed refusal
Release, 28
Repetitious questions, 15
Report Verification Documentation, 106
Reporting endorsement coverage, 81–82
Reporting of incident, timeliness of, 9
Request for Admission of Facts, 12–13
Request for Admission of Genuineness of Documents, 13
Reservation-of-rights letter, 90
Residents
   communication with attending staff, 46–47, 53
   and establishment of physician-patient relationship, 2, 56
   ethical considerations of, 56–58
   and informed consent, 39
   insurance of, 10
   lawsuits against, 8
   liability status of, 52–56
   and moral opposition to medical procedures, 57–58
   in outpatient/ambulatory care setting, 47
   professional liability insurance of, 80–84
      amount of, 82–83
      checklist for, 80–81
      future considerations for, 83–84
      restrictions on, 83
      types of, 81–82
   and settlements, 31–32
   and standards of care, 3–4, 52
   use of chaperones by, 48
Respondeat superior, 53, 55

Right-to-consent-to-settlement clause, in professional liability insurance, 87
Risk management
  in hospital setting, 44–47
  in outpatient/ambulatory care setting, 47–49
Risk manager
  and incident management, 9
  and settlements, 31
Risk purchasing groups, 85, 88
Risk retention groups, 85, 87–88
Rules and protocols, and risk management, 45

S

Security, of individually identifiable health information, 95–96
SEER Cancer Statistics Review 1973–1998, 63
Self-referral prohibitions, 97–98
Settlement, 27–32
  factors influencing decision for, 30–31
  at incident stage, 31
  insurance options for, 87, 89
  issues of, 29
  at lawsuit/formal claim stage, 31–32
Sexual misconduct, false charges of, 48
Sherwood v. Carter, 37
Shoulder dystocia, 63
Special damages, 6
Standard of care
  and breach of duty, 5
  establishment of, 4–5
  resident requirements for, 3–4, 52
  and risk management, 45

Standard of disclosure, 35–38
State laws, on informed consent, 38
State physician profiling, 106
Stillbirth, 61
Summation, 24
Summons, 9–10
Surcharging rating plans, 84

T

Tail coverage, 81–82
Tampering, with medical records, 11, 76
Technology
  and medical records, 74
  and privacy, 95
  and risk management, 45
Telephone conversations, notation in medical record, 74
Terminology, in medical records, 73
Testimony
  at deposition, 13–17
  at trial, 21–23
Timeliness
  of incident reporting, 9
  of medical records, 75–76
Transfer of patients
  in emergency room, 3
  interhospital, 92–95
Transport team, 94
Triage, attending staff–resident communication in, 47
Trial dates, 20–21
Trial stage, of medical professional liability lawsuit, 19–25

U

U.S. Department of Health and Human Services, and National Practitioner Data Bank, 104

V

Vacuum assisted delivery, 63
Vaginal birth after cesarean delivery (VBAC), 62
Vaginal delivery, operative, 62–63
VBAC. *See* Vaginal birth after cesarean delivery
Verdict, 23–25
Vicarious liability, 53–55

W

Witness
  pretrial preparation of, 20–22
  trial testimony of, 21